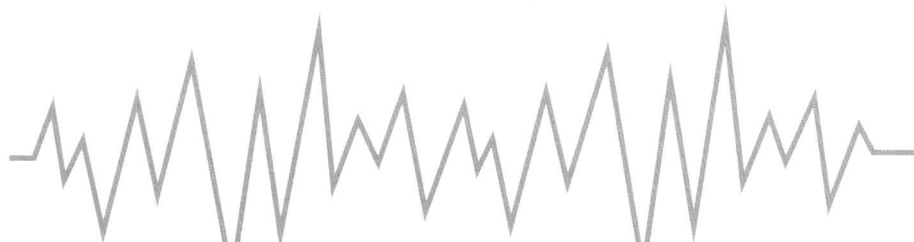

临床实用心电图

实例分析与解读（中英对照）

Frank G. Yanowitz 著

王绍军　刘巍 编译

周玉杰 审校

THE MASTERY
OF ECG INTERPRETATION

中南大学出版社
www.csupress.com.cn

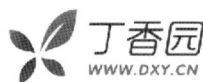

丁香园
WWW.DXY.CN

图书在版编目（ＣＩＰ）数据

临床实用心电图实例分析与解读：中英对照／（美）亚诺威（Yanowitz，F. G.）著；王绍军，刘巍编译． --长沙：中南大学出版社，2014.8
ISBN 978 - 7 - 5487 - 1186 - 5

Ⅰ.临…　Ⅱ.①亚…②王…③刘…　Ⅲ.心电图—图解
Ⅳ.R540.4 -64

中国版本图书馆 CIP 数据核字（2014）第 204635 号

临床实用心电图实例分析与解读

Frank G. Yanowitz　著

王绍军　刘巍　编译

□责任编辑　李　娴　孙娟娟
□责任印制　易红卫
□出版发行　中南大学出版社
　　　　　　社址：长沙市麓山南路　　　　邮编：410083
　　　　　　发行科电话：0731 - 88876770　　传真：0731 - 88710482
□印　　装　长沙鸿和印务有限公司

□开　　本　720×1000　B5　□印张 15　□字数 294 千字
□版　　次　2014 年 10 月第 1 版　□2017 年 12 月第 3 次印刷
□书　　号　ISBN 978 - 7 - 5487 - 1186 - 5
□定　　价　38.00 元

INTRODUCTION TO ECG INTERPRETATION

Frank G. Yanowitz, MD

Professor of Medicine

University of Utah School of Medicine

Director, IHC ECG Services

LDS Hospital & Intermountain Medical Center

Salt Lake City, Utah

frank. yanowitz@ imail. org

IHC(Intermountain Healthcare)是美国犹他州一个非盈利性质的、大型的、由多家医院、医生以及保险程序组成的健康机构。

LDS Hospital(Latter-Day-Saints Hospital)是 IHC 之中的一家医院。

前　言

这本书是献给 Alan E. Lindsay 博士 (1923—1987)，一位心电图专家、老师、朋友、导师和同事。本书中许多精彩的心电图分析、诊断策略和精华均来自于 Alan E. Lindsay 博士个人毕生收藏的心电图宝库。多年来，这些心电图一直用于训练医学生、护士、住院医师、心脏病研究员和在狄他州盐湖城工作的医生们。当然，这些心电图也被经常用于许多国家和地区的各类医学会议，非常实用和简洁易懂，深受欢迎。

很荣幸这本书能够翻译成中文并出版以纪念和缅怀 Alan E. Lindsay 博士的教学和他那伟大的爱。

Alan E. Lindsay 博士
一位颇具风度、有影响力的老师

读过或学过心电图的医生会经常发现，有些心电图的诊断标准和心电图术语，许多书本上的描述并不一致，老师教得也不完全一样。比如心室肥大的诊断标准，宽、窄 QRS 心动过速的鉴别等，各家说法不一。本书的目的就是希望统一心电图的诊断标准，规范心电图的术语。尽管最近的心电图学已经包含了一部分新的诊断概念，但还是需要在世界范围内对其进行广泛地交流和比较。重要的是，我们需要认识和真正掌握心电图诊断技能。要充分利用这个临床医学最有用的工具之一，只能靠获得大量的阅读心电图的经验后，将具有相关的病理特征的心电图与临床病人的实际情况相结合，才能作出准确的判断。这就是 Alan E. Lindsay 教授的精髓所在。

这本书列出了步进式心电图的判读方法(见第二节)。初学者应该按顺序学习。其他人可以选择任何他们感兴趣的章节。希望所有的读者最后都能留下一些热爱和喜欢心电图的体会，与我和 Alan E. Lindsay 教授共同分享。

本书仅供您参考。所有的材料都是如上所述所提供，关于资料的精度和操作性不能作任何保证。您阅读本书请接受所有使用本文的风险，并信赖本文包含的内容。

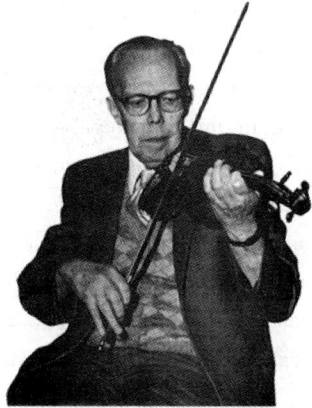

编译者

PREFACE

This booklet is dedicated to the memory of Alan E. Lindsay, MD (1923—1987) master teacher of electrocardiography, friend, mentor, and colleague. Many of the excellent ECG tracings illustrated in this learning program are from Dr. Lindsay's personal collection of ECG treasures. For many years these ECG's have been used in the training of medical students, nurses, house staff physicians, cardiology fellows, and practicing physicians in Salt Lake City, Utah as well as at many regional and national medical meetings.

Dr. Alan Lindsay:
A Teacher of Substance and Style

It is an honor to be able to provide this booklet as well as an interactive ECG website on the Internet in recognition of Dr. Lindsay's great love for teaching and for electrocardiography: http: //library. med. utah. edu/kw/ecg. This document and the ECG website offer an introduction to clinical electrocardiography.

ECG terminology and diagnostic criteria often vary from book to book and from one teacher to another. In this document an attempt has been made to conform to standardized terminology and criteria, although new diagnostic concepts derived from the recent ECG literature have been included in some of the sections. Finally, it is important to recognize that the mastery of ECG interpretation, one of the most useful clinical tools in medicine, can only occur if one acquires considerable experience in reading ECG's and correlating the specific ECG findings with the pathophysiology and clinical status of the patient.

The sections in this booklet are organized in the same order as the recommended step-wise approach to ECG interpretation outlined in Section 2. Beginning students should first go through the sections in the order in which they are presented. Others may choose to explore topics of interest in any order they wish. It is hoped that all students will be left with some of the love of electrocardiography shared by Dr. Lindsay.

The materials presented in the "Introduction to ECG Interpretation" booklet are for your information only. All of the materials are provided "AS IS" and without any warranty, express, implied or otherwise, regarding the materials' accuracy or performance. You accept all risk of use of, and reliance on, the materials contained in the booklet.

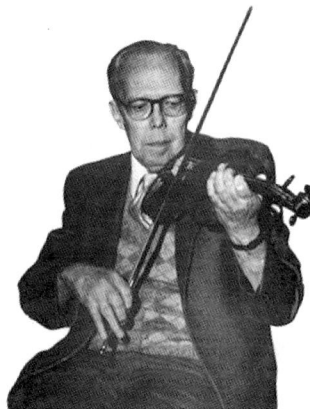

心电图基本能力

ECG 描记正常

- 正常 ECG

技术问题

- 导联错误
- 干扰

窦性心律/窦性心律失常

- 窦性心律
- 窦性心动过速
- 窦性心动过缓
- 窦性心律失常
- 窦性停搏
- 窦房阻滞，Ⅰ型
- 窦房阻滞，Ⅱ型

其他室上性心律失常

- 房性期前收缩（未下传）
- 房性期前收缩（正常传导）
- 房性期前收缩（伴差异传导）
- 异位房性心律或房速（单点）
- 多点房性心律或房速
- 心房纤颤
- 心房扑动
- 交界性期前收缩
- 交界性逸搏及交界性逸搏心律
- 加速性交界性逸搏心律
- 交界性心动过速
- 阵发性室上性心动过速

室性心律失常

- 室性期前收缩
- 室性逸搏及室性逸搏心律

- 室性心动过速（单型）
- 室性心动过速（多型或尖端扭转型室速）
- 心室颤动

房室传导

- 1 度房室传导阻滞
- 2 度Ⅰ型房室传导阻滞（文氏型）
- 2 度Ⅱ型房室传导阻滞（莫氏型）
- 高度房室传导阻滞
- 3 度房室传导阻滞（伴交界性逸搏心律）
- 3 度房室传导阻滞（伴室性逸搏心律）
- 房室分离（逸搏）
- 房室分离（夺获）
- 房室分离（房室传导阻滞伴逸搏）

室内传导

- 完全性左束支传导阻滞（持续或一过性）
- 不完全性左束支传导阻滞
- 完全性右束支传导阻滞（持续或一过性）
- 不完全性右束支传导阻滞
- 左前分支阻滞（LAFB）
- 左后分支阻滞（LPFB）
- 非特异性室内传导延缓（IVCD）
- 预激综合征（WPW）

QRS 电轴与电压

- 电轴右偏（+90°至+180°）
- 电轴左偏（-30°至-90°）
- 奇异电轴（-90°至-180°）
- 不确定的电轴
- 肢体导联低电压（<0.5 mV）

- 胸导联低电压(<1.0 mV)

肥厚/增大

- 左房增大
- 右房增大
- 双房增大
- 左室肥大
- 右室肥大
- 双室肥大

ST-T异常，U波异常

- 早期复极(正常变异)
- 非特异性ST-T异常
- ST段抬高(透壁性损伤)
- ST段抬高(心包炎)
- 对称性T波倒置
- 超急性T波
- 显著直立的U波
- U波倒置
- Q-T间期延长

心肌梗死(急性，近期，陈旧)

- 前壁梗死
- 下后壁梗死

- 后壁梗死
- 前间壁梗死
- 前壁梗死
- 前侧壁梗死
- 广泛前壁梗死
- 高侧壁梗死
- 非Q波梗死
- 右室梗死

临床问题

- 慢性阻塞性肺疾病
- 低血钾
- 高血钾
- 低钙血症
- 高钙血症
- 地高辛作用
- 地高辛中毒
- 中枢神经系统病变

起搏ECG

- 心房起搏心律
- 心室起搏心律
- 房室顺序起搏心律

Basic Competency in Electrocardiography

NORMAL TRACING

- Normal ECG

TECHNICAL PROBLEM

- Lead misplaced
- Artifact

SINUS RHYTHMS/ARRHYTHMIAS

- Sinus rhythm
- Sinus tachycardia
- Sinus bradycardia
- Sinus Arrhythmia
- Sinus arrest or pause
- Sinoatrial block, type I
- Sinoatrial block, type II

OTHER SV ARRHYTHMIAS

- PAC's (nonconducted)
- PAC's (conducted normally)
- PAC's (conducted with aberration)
- Ectopic atrial rhythm or tachycardia (unifocal)
- Multifocal atrial rhythm or tachycardia
- Atrial fibrillation
- Atrial flutter
- Junctional prematures
- Junctional escapes or rhythms
- Accelerated Junctional rhythms
- Junctional tachycardia
- Paroxysmal supraventricular tachycardia

VENTRICULAR ARRHYTHMIAS

- PVC's

- Ventricular escapes or rhythm
- Accelerated ventricular rhythm
- Ventricular tachycardia (uniform)
- Ventricular tachycardia (polymorphous or torsades)
- Ventricular fibrillation

AV CONDUCTION

- 1st degree AV block
- Type I 2nd degree AV block (Wenckebach)
- Type II 2nd degree AV block (Mobitz)
- AV block, advanced (high grade)
- 3rd degree AV block (junctional escape rhythm)
- 3rd degree AV block (ventricular escape rhythm)
- AV dissociation (default)
- AV dissociation (usurpation)
- AV dissociation (AV block)

INTRAVENTRICULAR CONDUCTION

- Complete LBBB, fixed or intermittent
- Incomplete LBBB
- Complete RBBB, fixed or intermittent
- Incomplete RBBB
- Left anterior fascicular block (LAFB)
- Left posterior fascicular block (LPFB)
- Nonspecific IV conduction delay (IVCD)
- WPW preexcitation pattern

QRS AXIS AND VOLTAGE

- Right axis deviation ($+90°$ to $+180°$)
- Left axis deviation ($-30°$ to $-90°$)

▶ 1

- Bizarre axis ($-90°$ to $-180°$)
- Indeterminate axis
- Low voltage frontal plane (<0.5 mV)
- Low voltage precordial (<1.0 mV)

HYPERTROPHY/ENLARGEMENTS

- Left atrial enlargement
- Right atrial enlargement
- Biatrial enlargement
- Left ventricular hypertrophy
- Right ventricular hypertrophy
- Biventricular hypertrophy

ST – T, AND U ABNORMALITIES

- Early repolarization (normal variant)
- Nonspecific ST – T abnormalities
- ST elevation (transmural injury)
- ST elevation (pericarditis pattern)
- Symmetrical T wave inversion
- Hyperacute T waves
- Prominent upright U waves
- U wave inversion
- Prolonged QT interval

MI PATTERNS (acute, recent, old)

- Interior MI
- Inferoposterior MI

- Inferoposterolateral MI
- Posterior MI
- Anteroseptal MI
- Anterior MI
- Anterolateral MI
- Extensive anterior MI
- High lateral MI
- Non Q-wave MI
- Right ventricular MI

CLINICAL DISORDERS

- Chronic pulmonary disease pattern
- Suggests hypokalemia
- Suggests hyperkalemia
- Suggests hypocalcemia
- Suggests hypercalcemia
- Suggests digoxin effect
- Suggests digoxin toxicity
- Suggests CNS disease

PACEMAKER ECG

- Atrial-paced rhythm
- Ventricular paced rhythm
- AV sequential paced rhythm
- Failure to capture (atrial or ventricular)
- Failure to inhibit (atrial or ventricular)
- Failure to pace (atrial or ventricular)

目　录

TABLE OF CONTENTS

Basic Competency in Electrocardiography

(Modified from: ACC/AHA Clinical Competence Statement, JACC 2001; 38: 2091)

In 2001 a joint committee of the American College of Cardiology and the American Heart Association published a list of ECG diagnoses considered to be important for developing basic competency in ECG interpretation. This list is illustrated on the following page and is also illustrated on the website with links to examples or illustrations of the specific ECG diagnosis. Students of electrocardiography are encouraged to study this list and become familiar with the ECG recognition of these diagnoses. Most of the diagnoses are illustrated in this document.

解读心电图的基本能力

(修改自: ACC/AHA 临床能力解读，JACC 2001; 38: 2091)

2001 年，美国心脏病学会（ACC）和美国心脏病协会（AHA）联合发表了一系列有关心电图诊断和临床能力评估的内容，认为心电图诊断能力是临床医生必须提高的基本技能，也鼓励医学生学习这些内容，并掌握心电图的诊断。这些内容本书在后面的章节中将详细陈述。

1 THE STANDARD 12 LEAD ECG

The standard 12-lead electrocardiogram is a representation of the heart's electrical activity recorded from electrodes on the body surface. This section describes the basic components of the ECG and the standard lead system used to record the ECG tracings.

The diagram illustrates ECG waves and intervals as well as standard time and voltage measures on the ECG paper.

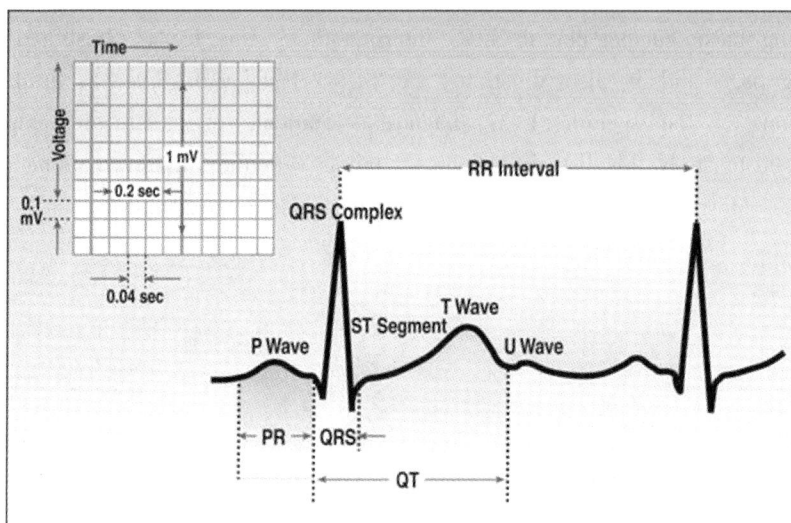

Fig. 1 – 1

1.1 ECG WAVES AND INTERVALS—What do they mean?

(1) P wave: sequential depolarization of the right and left atria

(2) QRS complex: right and left ventricular depolarization

(3) ST – T wave: ventricular repolarization

(4) U wave: an electrical-mechanical event at beginning of diastole

(5) PR interval: time interval from onset of atrial depolarization(P wave) to onset of ventricular muscle depolarization (QRS complex)

(6) QRS duration: duration of ventricular muscle depolarization(width of the QRS complex)

(7) QT interval: duration of ventricular depolarization and repolarization

(8) PP interval: rate of atrial or sinus cycle

(9) RR interval: rate of ventricular cycle

1　标准 12 导联心电图

标准 12 导联心电图是 10 个电极在体表采集到的心脏电活动的记录。本章主要描述心电图的基本组成和 12 导联体系。

图 1 - 1 显示了心电图各波波形、各波间期以及测量心电图的标准电压和走纸时间。

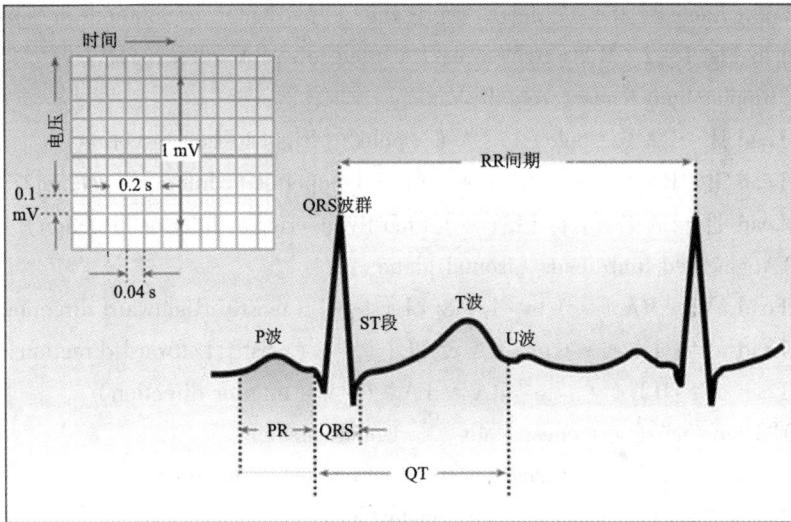

图 1 - 1

1.1　心电图中的各个波和间期代表什么?

(1) P wave(P 波):从右心房向左心房除极。

(2) QRS complex(QRS 波):右心室和左心室除极。

(3) ST - T wave(ST 段和 T 波):心室复极。

(4) U wave(U 波):舒张早期的电 - 机械事件。

(5) PR interval(PR 间期):从心房开始除极(P 波起始部)到心室肌开始除极(QRS 波起始部)的时间。

(6) QRS duration(QRS 间期):心室肌除极时间。

(7) QT interval(QT 间期):从心室开始除极到心室复极结束的时间。

(8) PP interval(PP 间期):窦性周期,2 个 P 波之间的时间。

(9) RR interval(RR 间期):室性周期,2 个 R 波之间的时间。

1.2 ORIENTATION OF THE 12-LEAD ECG

1.2.1 It is important to remember that the 12-lead ECG provides spatial information about the heart's electrical activity in 3 approximately orthogonal directions (think: X, Y, Z):

(1) Right − Left (X)

(2) Superior − Inferior (Y)

(3) Anterior − Posterior (Z)

1.2.2 Each of the 12 leads represents a particular orientation in space, as indicated in Fig. 1 −2 (RA = right arm; LA = left arm, LL = left leg):

(1) Bipolar limb leads (frontal plane):

- Lead Ⅰ: RA (− pole) to LA (+ pole) (Right-to-Left direction)
- Lead Ⅱ: RA (−) to LL (+) (mostlySuperior-to-Inferior direction)
- Lead Ⅲ: LA (−) to LL (+) (mostlySuperior-to-Inferior direction)

(2) Augmented limb leads (frontal plane):

- Lead aVR: RA (+) to [LA & LL] (−) (mostly Rightward direction)
- Lead aVL: LA (+) to [RA & LL] (−) (mostly Leftward direction)
- Lead aVF: LL (+) to [RA & LA] (−) (Inferior direction)

(3) "Unipolar" (+) chest leads (horizontal plane):

- Leads V1, V2, V3 (mostly Posterior-to-Anterior direction)
- Leads V4, V5, V6 (mostly Right-to-Left direction)

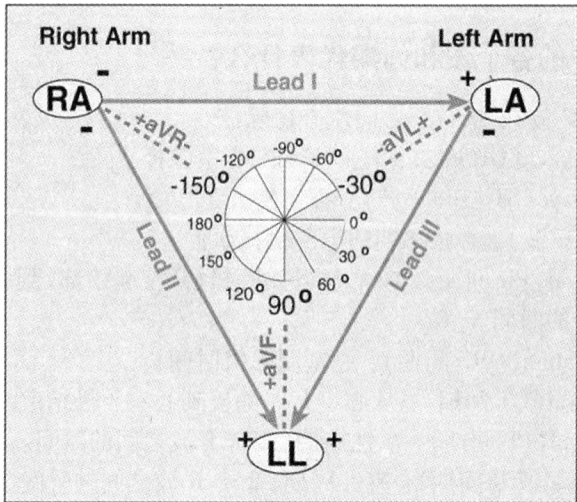

Fig. 1 −2

1.2   12 导联心电图的方向与定位

1.2.1   一定要知道 12 导联心电图提供的是一个关于心脏电活动的立体的空间概念，从 3 个正交的方向去定位(X，Y，Z 轴)：

(1)右－左（X）

(2)上－下（Y）

(3)前－后（Z）

1.2.2   12 导联中的每一个导联都代表了一个空间的方向，如图 1－2 所示（RA＝右上肢；LA＝左上肢，LL＝左下肢）。

(1)双极肢体导联（额面）：

- Ⅰ导联：RA(－极)到 LA(＋极)（由右向左方向）
- Ⅱ导联：RA(－)到 LL(＋)（由上向下方向）
- Ⅲ导联：LA(－)到 LL(＋)（从上到下方向）

(2)加压肢导联（额面）：

- aVR：RA(＋)到[LA&LL](－)（向右上方向）
- aVL：LA(＋)到[RA&LL](－)（向左上方向）
- aVF：LL(＋)到[RA&LA](－)（向下方向）

(3)胸导联(水平面)：

- V1，V2，V3(从后向前方向)
- V4，V5，V6(从右向左方向)

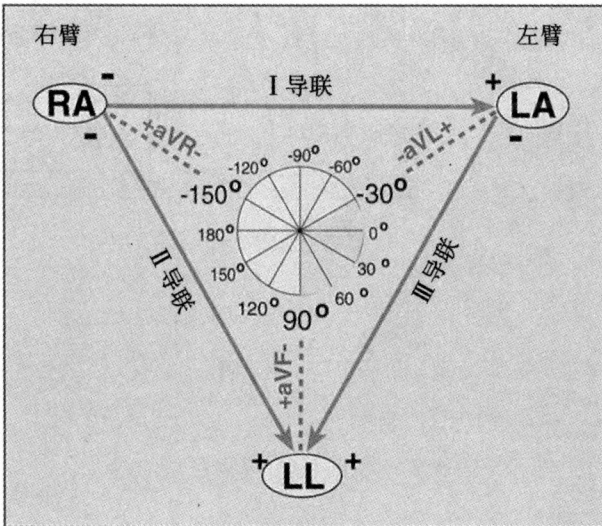

图 1－2

Behold: Einthoven's Triangle! Each of the 6 frontal plane or "limb" leads has a negative and positive pole (as indicated by the " + " and " – " signs). It is important to recognize that lead Ⅰ (and to a lesser extent aVL) are right-to-left in direction. Also, lead aVF (and to a lesser extent leads Ⅱ and Ⅲ) are superior-to-inferior in direction. The diagrams in Fig. 1 −3、Fig. 1 −4 further illustrate the frontal plane and chest lead hookup.

Note: the actual ECG waveform in each of the 6 limb leads varies from person to person depending on age, body size, gender, frontal plane QRS axis, presence or absence of heart disease, and many other variables. The precordial lead sites are illustrated below.

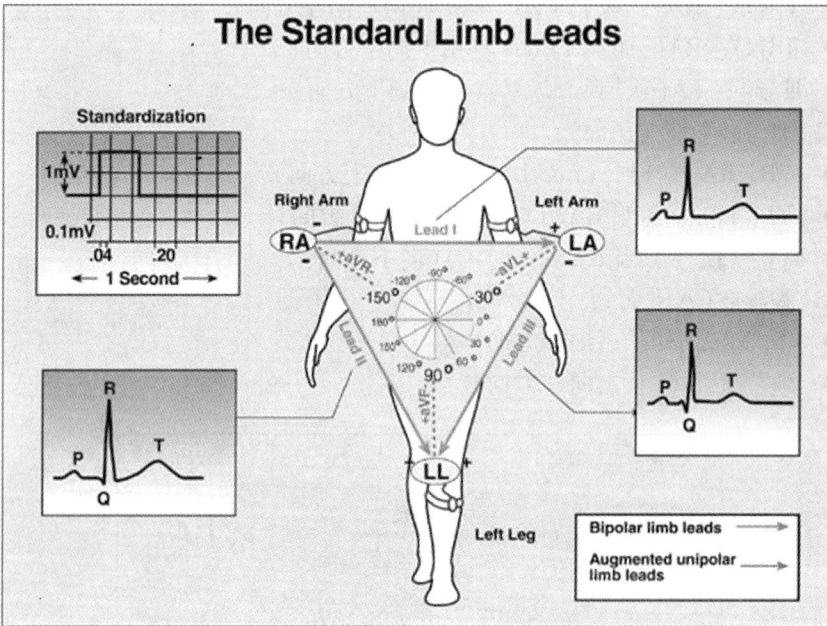

Fig. 1 −3

图1-2是著名的艾思文三角。额面肢体导联中的每一个导联都有一个阴极和一个阳极(见标记的"＋"和"－")。重点是Ⅰ导联(和L导联)方向是从右向左,Ⅱ和Ⅲ导联(和F导联)从上向下。图1-3、图1-4将进一步描述额面和胸前导联。

注:Ⅰ、Ⅱ、Ⅲ导联为双极导联,aVR、aVL、aVF为单极加压导联,V1～V8电极为胸前导联。

注意:实际上每个人每一个导联的心电图波形都是不同的,取决于年龄、性别、躯体大小,以及有无心脏病等诸多因素。胸前导联的位置如图1-3、图1-4所示。

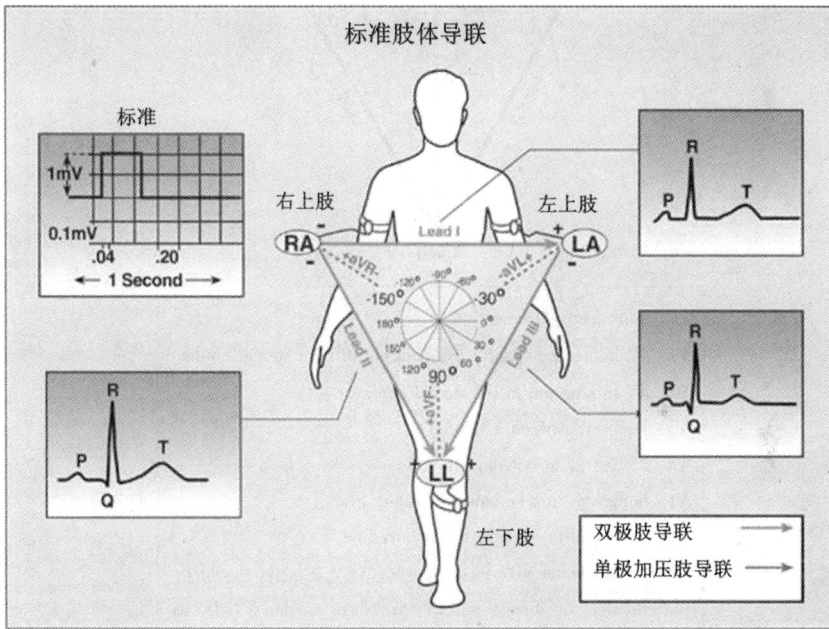

图1-3

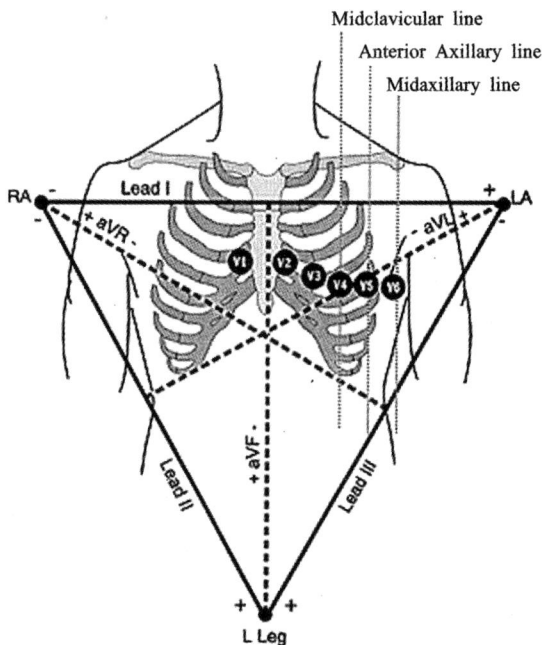

Midclavicular line
Anterior Axillary line
Midaxillary line

Precordial lead placement

V1: 4th intercostal space (IS) adjacent to right sternal border

V2: 4th IS adjacent to left sternal border

V3: Halfway between V2 and V4

V4: 5th IS, midclavicular line

V5: horizontal to V4; anterior axillary line

V6: horizontal to V4 − 5; midaxillary line

(Note: in women with large breasts, V4 − 6 leads should be placedunder the breast surface as close to the 5th IS as possible)

Fig. 1 − 4

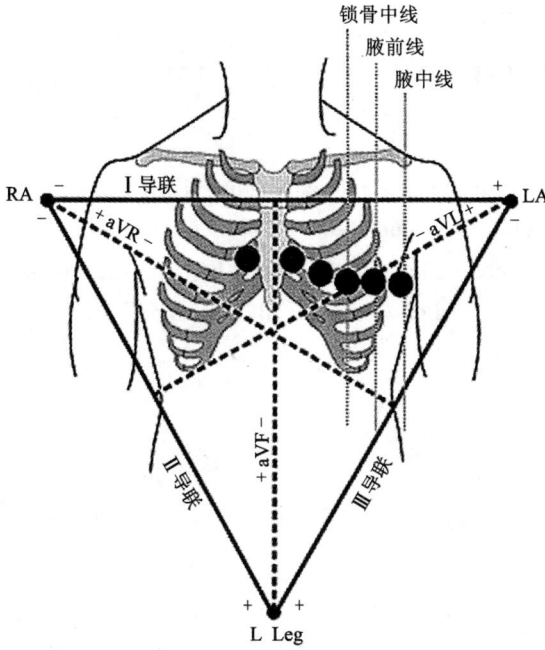

图 1-4

体表电极位置

V_1：第 4 肋间胸骨右缘

V_2：第 4 肋间胸骨左缘

V_3：V_2 及 V_4 导联之间（中点处）

V_4：第 5 肋间，左锁骨中线上

V_5：第 5 肋间，左腋前线上

V_6：第 5 肋间，V_4、V_5 之间，左腋中线上

2 A "METHOD" OF ECG INTERPRETATION

This "method" is recommended when reading 12-lead ECG's. Like the approach to doing a physical exam, it is important to follow a standardized sequence of steps in order to avoid missing subtle abnormalities in the ECG tracing, some of which may have clinical importance. The 6 major sections in the "method" should be considered in the following order:

    (1) Measurements

    (2) Rhythm analysis

    (3) Conduction analysis

    (4) Waveform description

    (5) ECG interpretation

    (6) Comparison with previous ECG (if available)

2.1 MEASUREMENTS (usually made in frontal plane leads):

- Heart rate (state both atrial and ventricular rates, if different)
- PR interval (from beginning of P to beginning of QRS complex)
- QRS duration (width of most representative QRS)
- QT interval (from beginning of QRS to end of T)
- QRS axis in frontal plane (see "How to Measure QRS Axis" on p14)

2.2 RHYTHM ANALYSIS:

- State the basic rhythm (e. g. , "normal sinus rhythm", "atrial fibrillation", etc.)
- Identify additional rhythm events if present (e. g. , "PVC's", "PAC's", etc)
- Remember that arrhythmias may originate in the atria, AV junction, and ventricles

2.3 CONDUCTION ANALYSIS:

"Normal" conduction implies normal sino-atrial (SA), atrio-ventricular (AV), and intraventricular (IV) conduction.

The following conduction abnormalities are to be identified if present:

2 阅读心电图的方法

建议用下面的方法阅读心电图。像体格检查一样，阅读心电图要按照标准的顺序和步骤进行，以免漏掉心电图中某些细微的异常，其中有的异常可能具有重要的临床意义。该方法主要有如下 6 个方面：

(1)测量
(2)节律分析
(3)传导分析
(4)波形分析
(5)心电图诊断
(6)与前图比较(如果可能)

2.1 测量(通常用于额面导联)

- 心率(包括心房率和心室率，两者是否相同)
- PR 间期[从心房开始除极(P 波)到心室肌开始除极(QRS 波)的时间]
- QRS 间期(最具代表性的 QRS 的宽度)
- QT 间期(从 QRS 起始到 T 波结束)
- QRS 额面电轴(如何测量 QRS 电轴，见 P15)

2.2 节律分析

- 描述基本节律(例如"正常窦性心律""心房纤颤"等)。
- 识别额外的节律事件[如室性期前收缩(PVC's)，房性期前收缩(PAC's)等]
- 牢记心律失常可以来自心房、房室结和心室。

2.3 传导分析

"正常"传导意味正常窦－房，房－室，以及心室内传导。应能够识别出下列传导异常：

- 2nd degree SA "exit" block (type Ⅰ, type Ⅱ, or uncertain)
- 1st, 2nd (type Ⅰ or type Ⅱ), and 3rd degree AV block
- Ⅳ blocks: bundle branch, fascicular, and nonspecific blocks
- Exit blocks are blocks just distal to the sinus or an ectopic pacemaker site

2.4 WAVEFORM DESCRIPTION:

Carefully analyze each of the 12-leads for abnormalities of the waveforms in the order in which they appear: P-waves, QRS complexes, ST segments, T waves, and... Don't forget the U waves.

- P waves: are they too wide, too tall, look funny (i. e., are they ectopic), etc. ?
- QRS complexes: look for pathologic Q waves, abnormal voltage, etc.
- ST segments: look for abnormal ST elevation and/or depression.
- T waves: look for abnormally inverted T waves or unusually tall T waves.
- U waves: look for prominent or inverted U waves.

2.5 ECG INTERPRETATION

This is the conclusion of the above analyses. Interpret the ECG as "Normal", or "Abnormal". Occasionally the term "borderline" is used if unsure about the significance of certain findings or for minor changes. List all abnormalities. Examples of "abnormal" statements are:

- Inferior MI, probably acute
- Old anteroseptal MI
- Left anterior fascicular block (LAFB)
- Left ventricular hypertrophy (LVH)
- Right atrial enlargement (RAE)
- Nonspecific ST – T wave abnormalities
- Specific rhythm abnormalities such as atrial fibrillation

Example of a 12-lead ECG interpretation (see below ECG tracing in Fig. 2 – 1):
HR = 67 bpm; PR = 0.18 s; QRS = 0.09 s; QT = 0.40 s; QRS axis = − 50° (left axis deviation).

Normal sinus rhythm; normal SA, AV, and Ⅳ conduction; rS waves in leads Ⅱ, Ⅲ, aVF (this means small r waves and large S waves); SⅢ > SⅡ.

Interpretation: Abnormal ECG: Left anterior fascicular block

- 2 度窦房传导阻滞(Ⅰ型,Ⅱ型或未确定)。
- 1 度,2 度(Ⅰ型或Ⅱ型),以及 3 度房室传导阻滞。
- 室内阻滞:束支,分支,以及非特异性传导阻滞。
- 传出阻滞,指窦性或异位起搏点的传导阻滞。

2.4 波形分析

仔细认真分析 12 导联中的每一个波形,发现异常波形。按顺序分析 P 波,QRS 波,ST 段,T 波,而且不要忘记 U 波。

- P 波:是否太宽,太高,看上去很奇怪(如,是异位 P 波?)等。
- QRS 波:找寻病理性 Q 波,电压异常等。
- ST 段:注意异常的 ST 抬高和(或)压低。
- T 波:注意异常倒置的 T 波或异常高大的 T 波。
- U 波:注意明显的或倒置的 U 波。

2.5 心电图诊断

这是通过上述分析后得出的结论。诊断该心电图"正常"或者"不正常",如果不确定某些微小改变的意义,可偶尔用"边缘"这个术语。例如"异常"的描述是:

- 下壁心肌梗死,可能急性。
- 陈旧性前间壁心肌梗死。
- 左前分支阻滞(LAFB)。
- 左心室肥大(LVH)。
- 右心房大(RAE)。
- 非特异性 ST‐T 改变。
- 特异性节律异常如心房纤颤。

12 导联心电图读图举例(见图 2‐1):

HR = 67 次/min;PR = 0.18 s;QRS = 0.09 s;QT = 0.40 s;QRS 电轴 = ‐50°(电轴左偏)。

正常窦性心律;正常窦房、房室和室内传导;Ⅱ,Ⅲ,aVF 为 rS(小 r 波和大 S 波);SⅢ > SⅡ。

读图诊断:异常心电图:左前分支阻滞(LAFB)

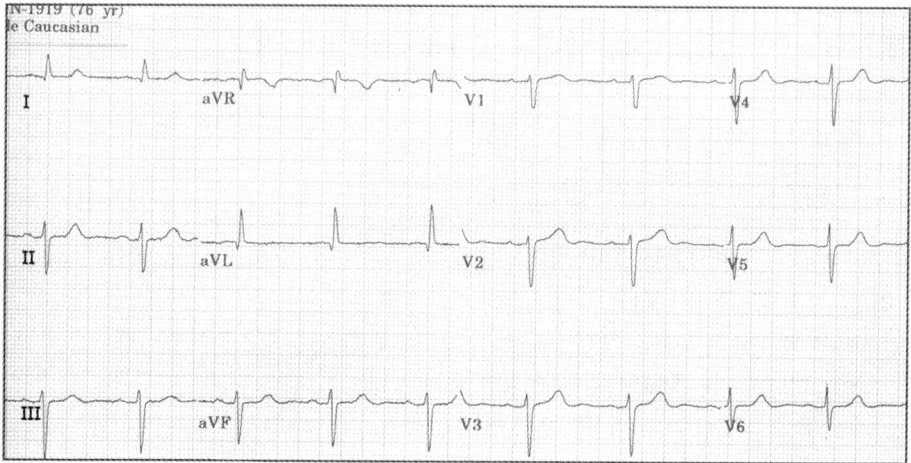

Fig. 2 – 1

2.6 COMPARISON WITH PREVIOUS ECG

If there is a previous ECG in the patient's file, the current ECG should be compared with it to see if any significant changes have occurred. These changes may have important implications for clinical management decisions.

2.6.1 HOW TO MEASURE THE QRS AXIS

The frontal plane QRS axis represents the average direction of ventricular depolarization forces in the frontal plane. As such this measure can inform the ECG reader of changes in the sequence of ventricular activation (e. g. , left anterior fascicular block), or it can be an indicator of myocardial damage (e. g. , inferior myocardial infarction). Determination of the QRS axis requires knowledge of the direction of the six individual frontal plain ECG leads. Einthoven's triangle enables us to visualize this.

In Fig. 2 – 3 the normal range is shaded gray (– 30° to + 90°). In the adult left axis deviation (i. e. , superior, leftward arrow) is defined from – 30° to – 90°, and right axis deviation (i. e. , inferior, rightward arrow) is defined from + 90° to + 180°. From – 90° to ± 180° is very unusual and may be due to lead placement error.

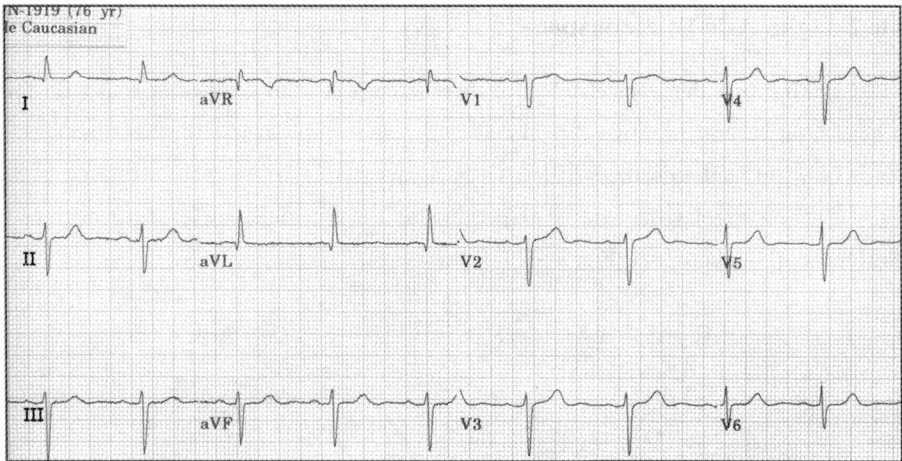

图 2 - 1

2.6 与以前的心电图比较

如果该患者病例档案中有以前的心电图,应该和以前的心电图进行比较,看两个心电图之间有没有明显的改变,如果有,这个变化具有重要的临床意义。

2.6.1 如何测量 QRS 电轴

额面 QRS 电轴代表心室除极在额面的方向,这一测量可以给我们提示心室电活动的顺序是否发生了改变(如左前分支阻滞),或提示存在心肌损害(如下壁心肌梗死)。QRS 电轴的判定需要知道额面心电图 6 个导联中每一个导联的方向,艾思文三角使其更加形象。

正常心电轴的范围是:-30°至 +90°,见图 2 - 3 中灰色阴影部分。成人电轴左偏(向上,向左的箭头)定义在 -30°至 -90°,电轴右偏(向下,向右的箭头)定义在 +90°至 +180°。从 -90°至 ±180°是非常罕见的,常常是由于导联电极位置错误所致。

2.6.2   QRS Axis Determination:

(1) First find the isoelectriclead if there is one; it's the lead with equal QRS forces in both positive and negative direction (i. e. , above and below the baseline). Often this is also the lead with the smallest QRS complex.

(2) The correct QRS axis is perpendicular (i. e. , right angle or 90 degrees) to that lead's orientation (see Fig. 2 – 2).

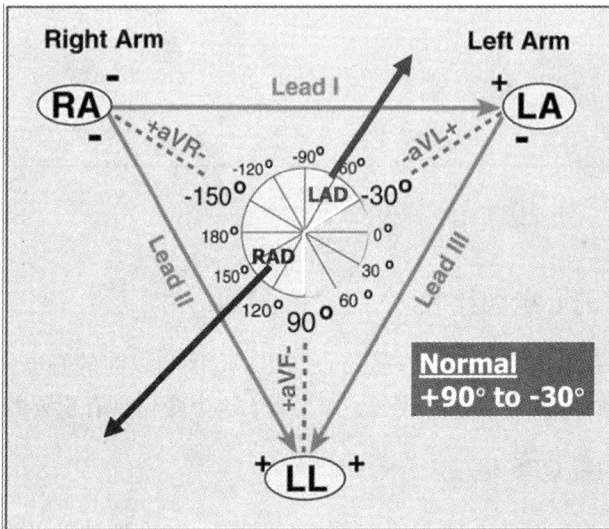

Fig. 2 – 2

(3) Since there are two possible perpendiculars for each isoelectric lead, one must chose the one that best fits the direction of the QRS forces in other ECG leads.

Table 2 – 1

Isoelectric Lead	More likely axis	Less likely axis
I	+90°	−90°
II	−30°	+150°
III	+30°	−150°
aVR	−60°	+120°
aVL	+60°	−120°
aVF	0	+／−180°

2.6.2　QRS 电轴的确定

(1)首先找出**等电位**导联(如果有);就是指在这个导联上的 QRS 波在基线上方的正向波幅与基线下方的负向波幅大小相等。通常在这个导联上的 QRS 波最小。

(2)QRS 电轴应该与该导联相垂直(或正交于等电位导联,呈 90°直角,见图 2 - 2)。

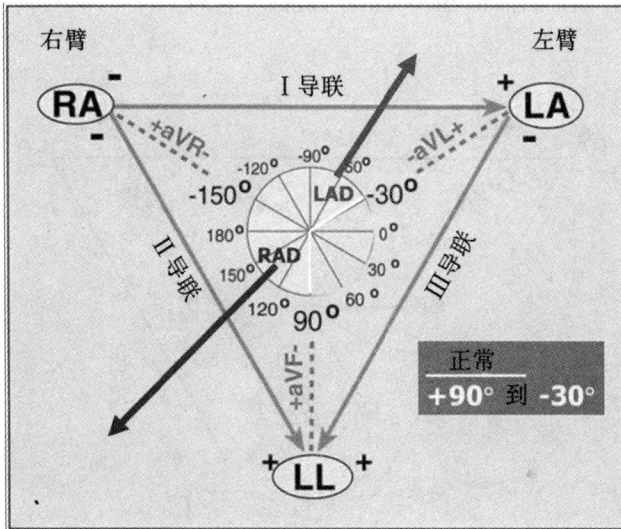

图 2 - 2

(3)每个导联都有两个可能的正交方向,我们必须在其他的 ECG 导联中选出最合适的 QRS 电轴方向。

表 2 - 1

等电位导联	最可能的电轴	最不可能的电轴
I	+90°	-90°
II	-30°	+150°
III	+30°	-150°
aVR	-60°	+120°
aVL	+60°	-120°
aVF	0°	+/-180°

(4) If there is no isoelectric lead, there are usually two leads that are nearly isoelectric, and these are always 30° apart in Fig. 2 – 2. Find the perpendiculars for each lead and chose an approximate QRS axis within the 30° range.

(5) Occasionally each of the 6 frontal plane leads is small and/or isoelectric. An axis cannot be determined and is called indeterminate. This is a normal variant.

2.6.3　Examples of QRS Axis Determination:

example 1.　An axis in thenormal range (−30° to +90°):

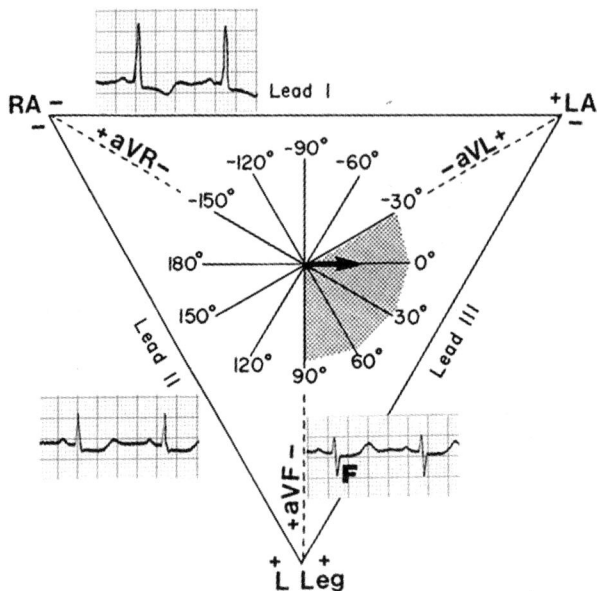

Fig. 2 – 3

Analysis (see Fig. 2 –3)

(1) Lead aVF is the isoelectric lead (equal forces positive and negative).

(2) The two perpendiculars to aVF are 0° and ±180°.

(3) Note that Lead I is all positive (i. e. , moving to the left).

(4) Therefore, of the two choices, the axis has to be 0°(arrow in Fig. 2 – 3).

（4）如果没有等电位的导联，通常会有两个接近等电位的导联，而且相距30°，见图2-2。找出这2个导联的正交方向并在这30°范围内选择一个大致的心电轴。

（5）偶见额面的6个导联都是小的QRS和/或等电位，使电轴无法确认，被称为不确定电轴，属正常变异。

2.6.3 下面是确定QRS电轴的实例

例1. 电轴正常范围（-30°至+90°）

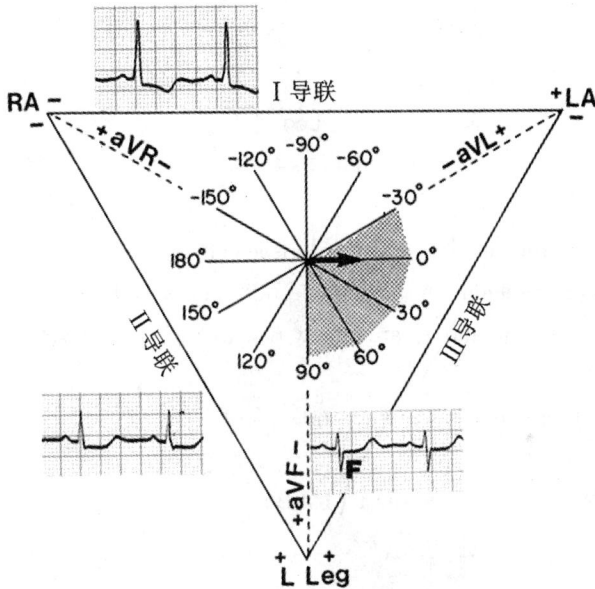

图2-3

分析

（1）aVF导联是等电位导联（正向波与负向波相等）。

（2）与aVF正交的是Ⅰ导联（0°和±180°）。

（3）注意Ⅰ导联QRS是正向波（电流从右流向左）。

（4）因此电轴指向0°（如图2-3中箭头所示）。

example 2. Left Axis deviation（LAD）：

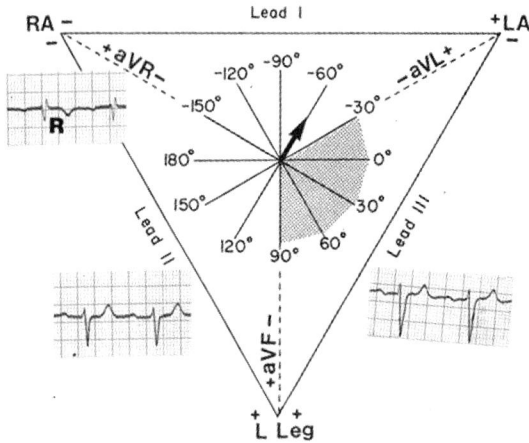

Fig. 2 – 4

Analysis

（1）Lead aVR is the smallest and nearly isoelectric.

（2）The two perpendiculars to aVR are −60° and +120°.

（3）Note that Leads Ⅱ and Ⅲ are mostly negative（i. e. , moving away from the + left leg）.

（4）The axis, therefore, has to be −60°（LAD）.

example 3. Right Axis Deviation（RAD）：

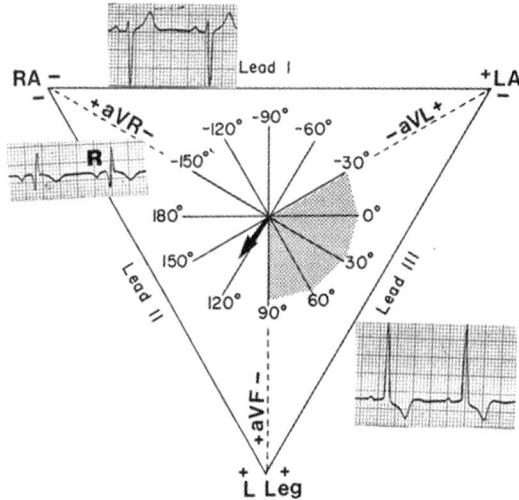

Fig. 2 – 5

例2. 电轴左偏（LAD）

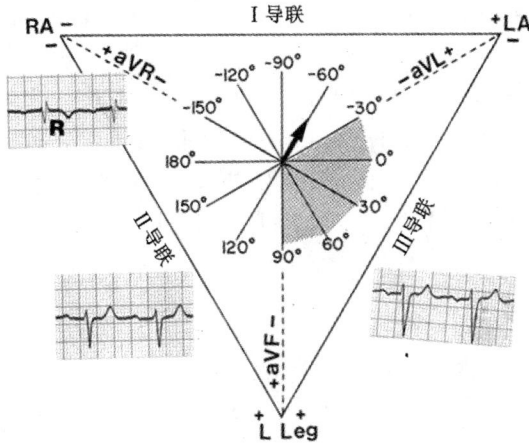

图2-4

分析

（1）aVR 导联 QRS 波最小而且接近等电位线。

（2）与 aVR 正交的方向分别是 -60°和 +120°。

（3）注意Ⅱ和Ⅲ大部分是负向波（电流从左下肢向上流动）。

（4）因此电轴指向左上 -60°（LAD）。

例3. 电轴右偏（RAD）

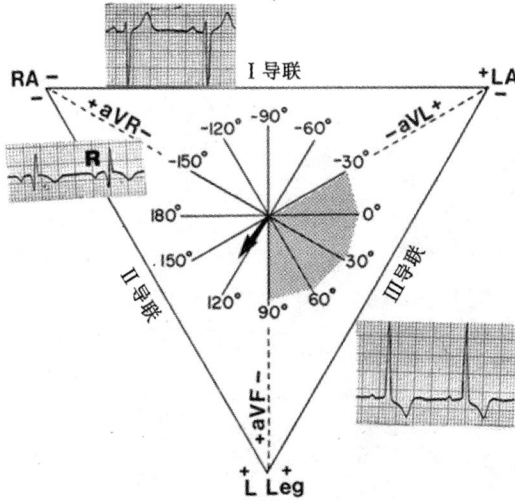

图2-5

Analysis

(1) Lead aVR is closest to being isoelectric (but slightly more positive than negative).

(2) The two perpendiculars to aVR are $-60°$ and $+120°$.

(3) Note that Lead Ⅰ is mostly negative; lead Ⅲ is mostly positive.

(4) Therefore the axis is close to $+120°$. Because aVR is slightly more positive, the axis is slightly beyond $+120°$ (i. e., closer to the positive right arm for aVR, about $+125°$).

分析

（1）aVR 最接近于等电位线（但是正向波略大于负向波）。

（2）正交于 aVR 的是 −60° 和 +120°。

（3）注意 I 大部分为负向波；III 大部分是正向波。

（4）因此电轴接近 +120°，因为 aVR 正向波略大于负向波，电轴应略超过 +120°（更接近右上肢，大约 +125°）。

3 CHARACTERISTICS OF THE NORMAL ECG

It is important to remember that there is a wide range of normal variation in the 12 lead ECG. The following "normal" ECG characteristics, therefore, are not absolute. It takes considerable ECG reading experience to discover all the normal variants. Only by following a structured "Method of ECG Interpretation" and correlating the various ECG findings with the patient's particular clinical status will the ECG become a valuable clinical tool.

3.1 Normal MEASUREMENTS (in adults)

(1) Heart Rate: 50 – 90 bpm (some ECG readers use 60 – 100 bpm)

(2) PR Interval: 0.12 – 0.20 s

(3) QRS Duration: 0.06 – 0.10 s

(4) QT Interval ($QT_c > 0.39$ s, < 0.45 s in men; > 0.39 s, < 0.46 s in women)

Poor Man's Guide to the upper limit of QT_c: HR = 70 bpm, $QT_c \leqslant 0.40$ s; for every 10 bpm increase above 70 bpm subtract 0.02 s, and for every 10 bpm decrease below 70 bpm add 0.02 s. For example:

$QT_c \leqslant 0.38$ s, HR = 80 bpm

$QT_c \leqslant 0.42$ s, HR = 60 bpm

(5) Frontal Plane QRS Axis: $+90°$ to $-30°$ (in the adult)

3.2 Normal RHYTHM

Normal sinus rhythm

3.3 Normal CONDUCTION

Normal Sino-Atrial (SA), Atrio-Ventricular (AV), and Intraventricular (IV) conduction

3.4 Normal WAVEFORM DESCRIPTION:

3.4.1 P Wave

It is important to remember that the P wave represents the sequential activation of the right and left atria, and it is common to see notched or biphasic P waves of right and left atrial activation.

3 正常心电图特征

12 导联心电图正常变异范围很大，因此下列"正常"心电图的特征并不是绝对的，要利用心电图的阅读经验去找出和发现所有的正常变异。只有遵循下列"心电图读图方法"的结构，以及把各种心电图所见与患者的特殊临床状态相结合才能使心电图成为有价值的临床工具。

3.1 成人 ECG 正常值

（1）心率：50 ~ 90 次/min（有的学者用 60 ~ 100 次/min）。

（2）PR 间期：0.12 ~ 0.20 s。

（3）QRS 间期：0.06 ~ 0.10 s。

（4）QT 间期（QT_c，男 > 0.39 s，< 0.45 s；女 > 0.39 s，< 0.46 s）。

QT 间期上限：心率为 70 次/min 时，QT_c ≤ 0.40 s；心率在 70 次/min 以上时，每增加 10 次/min 减去 0.02 s，心率在 70 次/min 以下时，每减慢 10 次/min，QT_c 增加 0.02 s。比如：

QT_c ≤ 0.38 s，心率为 80 次/min；

QT_c ≤ 0.42 s，心率为 60 次/min。

（5）额面 QRS 电轴：+90° 至 −30°（成人）。

3.2 正常节律

正常窦性心律。

3.3 正常传导

正常窦房（SA）、房室（AV）和室内（IV）传导。

3.4 正常波形描述

3.4.1 P 波

重点记住 P 波代表右心房和左心房的顺序兴奋，而且右心房和左心房活动经常可以见到有切迹的或者双向的 P 波。

(1) P duration < 0.12 s

(2) P amplitude < 2.5 mm

(3) Frontal plane P wave axis: 0° to +75° (i. e. , P must be up or + in Ⅰ and Ⅱ)

- May see notched P waves in frontal plane, and biphasic P (+/−) in V1

3.4.2 QRS Complex

The normal QRS represents the simultaneous activation of the right and left ventricles, although most of the QRS waveform is derived from the larger left ventricular musculature.

(1) QRS duration ≤ 0.10 s

(2) QRS amplitude is quite variable from lead to lead and from person to person. Two determinates of QRS voltages are:

- Size of the ventricular chambers (i. e. , the larger the chamber, the larger the voltage; often seen in young aerobic trained athletes)

- Proximity of chest electrodes to ventricular chamber (the closer, the larger the voltage; seen in tall, thin people)

(3) Frontal plane leads:

- The normal QRS axis range (+90° to −30°) implies that the QRS direction must always be positive (i. e. , up going) in leads Ⅰ and Ⅱ.

- Small "septal" q-waves are often seen in leads Ⅰ and aVL when the QRS axis is to thel eft of +60°, or in leads Ⅱ, Ⅲ, aVF when the QRS axis is to the right of + 60°.

(4) Precordial leads:

- Small r-waves begin in V1 or V2 and increase in size up to V5. The R-V6 is usually smaller than R-V5.

- In reverse, the s-waves begin in V6 or V5 and increase in size up to V2. S − V1 is usually smaller than S − V2.

- The usual transition from S > R in the right precordial leads to R > S in the left precordial leads is V3 or V4.

- Small normal "septal" q-waves may be seen in leads V5 and V6.

(1)P 波时间 <0.12 s。

(2)P 振幅(电压) <2.5 mm(0.25 mV)。

(3)额面 P 波电轴:0°至 +75°[如 P 波在 Ⅰ 和 Ⅱ 必须是直立(+)]。

(4)额面可以见到有切迹的 P 波,V1 可以见到双向 P 波(+/ −)。

3.4.2 QRS 波群

正常 QRS 波代表右心室和左心室的同步活动,但是大部分的 QRS 波源于大的左心室心肌。

(1)QRS 时间 ≤0.10 s。

(2)QRS 振幅(电压):在导联和导联之间,人与人之间有相当大的变异,其主要决定因素有两个:

- 心室大小(如,心室越大,电压越高;常见于年轻的有氧健身训练的运动员)。
- 电极与心腔的距离(距离越近,电压越大;见于瘦高的体型)。

(3)额面导联

- 正常的 QRS 电轴范围(+90°到 −30°)意味着在 Ⅰ 和 Ⅱ 导联中 QRS 的方向必须一直是正向(向上)。
- 当 QRS 电轴在 +60° 左侧时,在 Ⅰ 和 aVL 导联可见小的"间隔"q 波,当 QRS 电轴在 +60° 右侧时,在 Ⅱ,Ⅲ,aVF 导联也可以见到。

(4)胸前导联

- V1,V2 小 r 波然后逐渐增大为大的 R 波,一般 V5 最大,V6 略小于 V5。
- 而 S 波从 V6 或 V5 向 V2 方向逐渐加深,通常 S − V1 略小于 S − V2。
- 胸前导联一般在 V3 或 V4 处从 S > R 过渡到 R > S。
- V5 和 V6 可以见到小的"间隔"q 波。

3.4.3 ST Segment

In a sense, the term "ST segment" is a misnomer, because a discrete ST segment distinct from the T wave is often not seen. More frequently the ST – T wave is a smooth, continuous waveform beginning with the J-point (end of QRS), slowly rising to the peak of the T and followed by a more rapid descent to the isoelectric baseline or the onset of the U wave. This gives rise to asymmetrical T waves in most leads. The ST segment occurs during Phase 2 (the plateau) of the myocardial cell action potentials. In some normal individuals, particularly women, the T wave looks more symmetrical and a distinct horizontal ST segment is present.

The ST segment is oftenelevated above baseline in leads with large S waves (e. g., V2, V3), and the normal configuration is concave upward. ST segment elevation with concave upward appearance may also be seen in other leads; this is called the early repolarization pattern, and is often seen in young, male athletes (see an example of "early repolarization" in leads V4 ~ V6 in the ECG below). J-point elevation is often accompanied by a small J-wave in the lateral precordial leads. The physiologic basis for the J-wave is related to transient outward K^+ current during phase I of the epicardial and mid-myocardial cells, but not present in the subendocardial cells. Prominent J waves are can also be seen in hypothermia (also called Osborn waves).

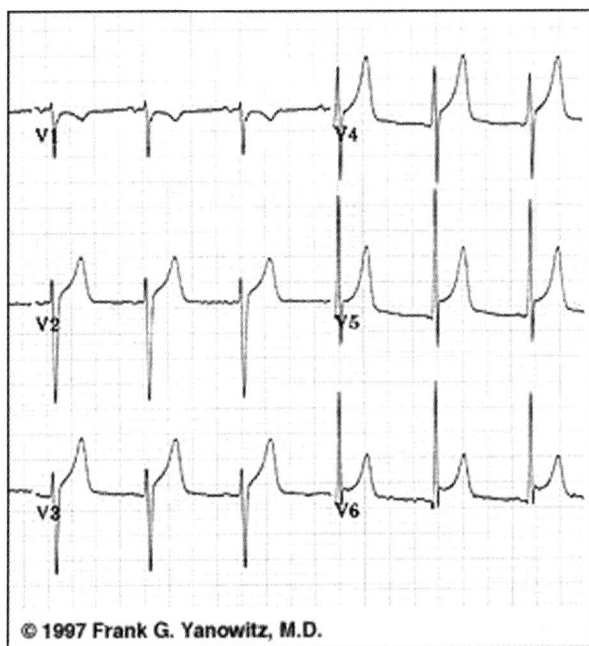

© 1997 Frank G. Yanowitz, M.D.

Fig. 3 – 1

3.4.3　ST 段

一般来说，术语"ST 段"是模糊的，因为常常很难区分 T 波起点。ST – T 波常常是平滑的、连续的、始于 J 点（QRS 终点），缓慢上升到 T 顶峰又快速下降到等电位线或 U 波起点，这导致了许多导联 T 波的非对称性。ST 段产生于心肌细胞动作电位的 2 相（平台期），某些正常人，尤其是女性可以表现为一个对称的 T 波和明显水平的 ST 段。

ST 段在 S 波较大的导联通常抬高到基线以上（如 V2、V3），而且正常情况下是凹面向上的抬高。ST 段凹面向上的抬高也可见其他导联，称**早期复极**，常见于年轻人和男运动员（图 3 – 1 的心电图中 V4 ~ V6 导联是一个"早期复极"）。在侧面胸前导联中可见到 J 点抬高并通常伴有一个小的 J 波。J 波产生的生理基础是与心外膜和中膜的心肌细胞（不包括心内膜下细胞）一过性 1 相 K^+ 外流有关。明显的 J 波也见于低体温（也称 Osborn 波）。

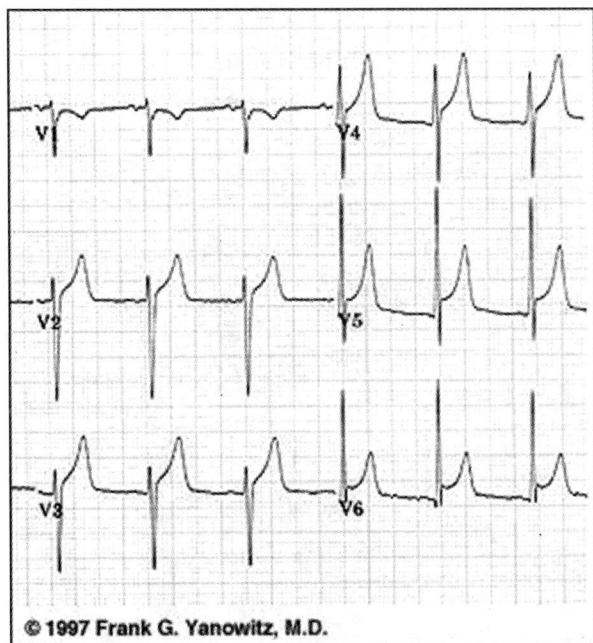

© 1997 Frank G. Yanowitz, M.D.

图 3 – 1

4　ECG MEASUREMENT ABNORMALITIES

4.1　PR Interval

(measured from beginning of P to beginning of QRS in the frontal plane)

4.1.1　Normal: 0.12 – 0.20 s

4.1.2　Differential Diagnosis of Short PR(<0.12 s)

(1)Preexcitation syndromes:

● WPW (Wolff-Parkinson-White) Syndrome: An accessory pathway (called the "Kent" bundle) connects the right atrium to the right ventricle or the left atrium to the left ventricle, and this permits early and slow activation of the ventricles (a delta wave) and a short PR interval (see Fig.4 – 1 for example).

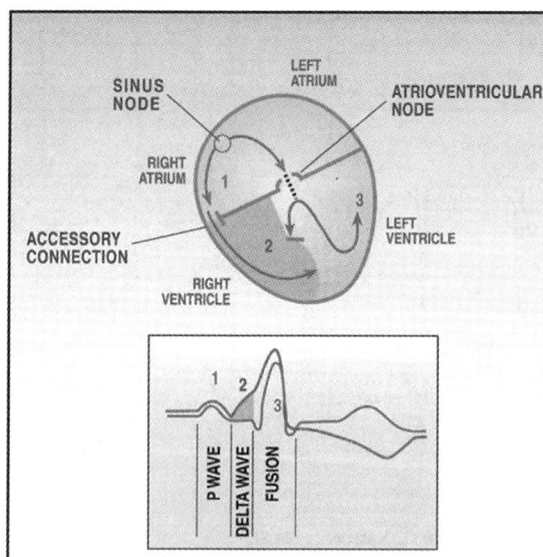

Fig.4 – 1

● LGL (Lown-Ganong-Levine) Syndrome: An AV nodal bypass track into the His bundle exists, and this permits early activation of the ventricles without a delta-wave because the ventricular activation sequence is unchanged; the PR interval, however, is shorter.

4　心电图测量异常

4.1　PR 间期（测量额面导联 P 波起始点到 QRS 起始点的时间）

4.1.1　正常值：0.12～0.20 秒（s）。

4.1.2　如果 PR 间期 <0.12 s，鉴别诊断包括：

（1）预激综合征

● WPW（Wolff-Parkinson-White）综合征：一个旁路（称"Kent"束）将右心房和右心室相连接或将左心房和左心室相连接，这导致了心室过早的缓慢的除极，产生 delta 波和一个短的 PR 间期（图 4-1）。

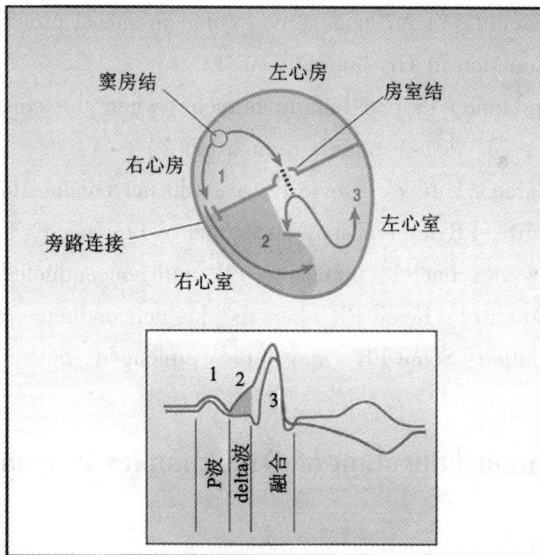

图 4-1

● LGL（Lown-Ganong-Levine）综合征：一个 AV 结的旁路绕过 AV 结直接与希氏束（His bundle）相连接，导致了心室性提前除极，但是没有 delta 波，因为心室除极的顺序没有改变，PR 间期却缩短了。

(2) AV Junctional Rhythms with retrograde atrial activation (inverted P waves in Ⅱ, Ⅲ, aVF) : Retrograde P waves may occur before the QRS complex (usually with a short PR interval) , within the QRS complex (i. e. , hidden from view) , or after the QRS complex (i. e. , in the ST segment) . It all depends upon the relative timing from the junctional focus antegrade into the ventricles vs. retrograde back to the atria.

(3) Ectopic atrial rhythms originating near the AV node (the PR interval is short because atrial activation originates closer to the AV node; the P wave morphology is different from the sinus P and may appear inverted in some leads) ; these are sometimes called "coronary sinus rhythms".

(4) Normal variant (PR 0. 10 – 0. 12 s) : seen in children and adolescents

4.1.3　Differential Diagnosis of Prolonged PR(>0. 20 s)

(1) First degree AV block (PR interval is usually constant from beat to beat) ; possible locations for the conduction delay include :
- Intra-atrial conduction delay (uncommon)
- Slowed conduction in AV node (most common site of prolonged PR)
- Slowed conduction in His bundle (rare)
- Slowed conduction in one bundle branch (when the contralateral bundle is totally blocked; i. e. , 1st degree bundle branch block)

(2) Second degree AV block (some P waves do not conduct to ventricles and are not followed by a QRS; PR interval may be normal or prolonged)
- Type Ⅰ (Wenckebach) : Increasing PR until nonconducted P wave occurs
- Type Ⅱ (Mobitz) : Fixed PR intervals plus nonconducted P waves

(3) AV dissociation : Some PR's may appear prolonged, but the P waves and QRS complexes are dissociated.

4.2　QRS Duration (duration of QRS complex in frontal plane) :

4.2.1　Normal : 0. 06 – 0. 10 s

4.2.2　Differential Diagnosis of Prolonged QRS Duration (>0. 10 s) :

(1) QRS duration 0. 10 – 0. 12 s
- Incompleteright or left bundle branch block
- Nonspecific intraventricular conduction delay (IVCD)
- Some cases of leftanterior or left posterior fascicular block

（2）AV 交界性心律伴有逆传导致心房除极（Ⅱ，Ⅲ，aVF 可见到倒置的 P 波）：逆传 P 可以出现在 QRS 之前（通常是短的 PR 间期），逆传 P 也可以在 QRS 波群中（如隐藏在 QRS 中看不到），或出现在 QRS 波群后（如出现在 ST 段上）。这取决于交界区起搏点前向传导到心室和逆传到心房的时间。

（3）距离房室结较近的异位房性节律（PR 间期缩短因为心房起搏点距离房室结近；P 波形态不同于正常窦性 P 波形态，而且可能在有些导联是倒置的；有时也叫"冠状窦节律"）。

（4）正常变异（PR 0.10 ~ 0.12 s）：可见于儿童和青少年。

4.1.3 PR 间期 >0.20 s 的鉴别诊断

（1）1 度房室传导阻滞（First degree AV block）：PR 间期恒定延长；传导延缓的部位可能在：
- 心房内传导延缓（不常见）。
- AV 结传导延缓（PR 延长的最常见部位）。
- 希氏束内传导延缓（少见）。
- 发生在一个束支的传导延缓（当对侧束支完全阻滞时，如 1st 度束支阻滞）。

（2）2 度房室传导阻滞（Second degree AV block）：有的 P 波不能传导到心室，P 波后没有 QRS；PR 间期可能是正常的或延长。
- Ⅰ型（文氏，Wenckebach）：PR 逐渐延长直到出现不能下传的 P 波。
- Ⅱ型（莫氏，Mobitz）：PR 固定不变加不能下传的 P 波。

（3）房室分离：有些 PR 可能延长，但是 P 波和 QRS 波群相互分离。

4.2 QRS 间期（额面 QRS 波群的时间）

4.2.1 正常：0.06 ~ 0.10 s。

4.2.2 QRS 时间延长（>0.10 s）的鉴别诊断

（1）QRS 时间 0.10 ~ 0.12 s
- 不完全的右或左束支传导阻滞。
- 非特异性室内传导延缓（IVCD）。
- 某些左前分支阻滞。

（2）QRS duration≥0.12 s

- Complete RBBB or LBBB
- Nonspecific IVCD
- Ectopic rhythms originating in the ventricles（e. g. , ventricular tachycardia, accelerated ventricular rhythm, pacemaker rhythm）

4.3　QT Interval

（measured from beginning of QRS to end of T wave in the frontal plane; corrected $QT = QT_c = $ measured $QT \div sq - root\ RR$ in seconds; Bazet's formula）

4.3.1　Normal QT is heart rate dependent（upper limit for $QT_c = 0.46$ sec）

4.3.2　Long QT Syndrome

LQTS（based on corrected QT_c: $QT_c \geqslant 0.45$ sec for males and $\geqslant 0.46$ sec in females is diagnostic for hereditary LQTS in the absence of other causes of long QT）:

This abnormality may have important clinical implications since it usually indicates a state of increased vulnerability to malignant ventricular arrhythmias, syncope, and sudden death. The prototype arrhythmia of the Long QT Interval Syndromes（LQTS）is Torsade-de-pointes, a polymorphic ventricular tachycardia characterized by varying QRS morphology and amplitude around the isoelectric baseline. Causes of LQTS include the following:

- Drugs（many antiarrhythmics, tricyclics, phenothiazines, and others）
- Electrolyte abnormalities（$\downarrow K^+$, $\downarrow Ca^{2+}$, $\downarrow Mg^{2+}$）
- CNS disease（especially subarachnoid hemorrhage, stroke, head trauma）
- Hereditary LQTS（at least 7 genotypes are now known）
- Coronary Heart Disease（some post-MI patients）
- Cardiomyopathy

4.3.3　Short QT Syndrome（$QT_c < 0.32$ sec）

Newly described hereditary disorder with increased risk of sudden　　　hmic death. The QT_c criteria are subject to change.

(2) QRS 时间≥0.12 s

- 完全性右束支或左束支传导阻滞。
- 非特异性室内传导延缓(IVCD)。
- 起源于心室的异位节律(如室性心动过速,加速性室性心律,起搏心律)。

4.3 QT 间期

(额面导联 QRS 起点到 T 波终点;校正的 QT = QT_c = QT ÷ $\sqrt{RR}$, Bazet's 公式)

4.3.1 正常 QT 取决于心率快慢(上限 QT_c = 0.46 s)

4.3.2 长 QT 综合征(LQTS)

基于校正的 QT_c,当男性 QT_c≥0.45 s,女性 QT_c≥0.46 s 时,如果没有导致 QT 延长的其他原因,可诊断为遗传性(家族性)长 QT 综合征。

这个异常具有重要的临床意义,因为这种状态很容易增加致死性室性心律失常的发生概率,甚至导致晕厥和猝死。长 QT 综合征(LQTS)所致的典型心律失常是尖端扭转型室性心动过速(Torsade-de-pointes),这是一种多型性的室性心动过速,以围绕等电线的 QRS 形态和幅度不断变化为特征。LQTS 原因如下:

- 药物(许多抗心律失常药,三环类,吩噻嗪类等)。
- 电解质紊乱(K^+↓,Ca^{2+}↓,Mg^{2+}↓)。
- 中枢神经系统疾病(特别是蛛网膜下隙出血、脑卒中、脑外伤)。
- 遗传性 LQTS(目前所知至少有 7 种基因型)。
- 冠心病(某些后壁心肌梗死患者)。
- 心肌病。

4.3.3 短 QT 综合征(QT_c<0.32 s)

新近报道,遗传问题可导致心律失常性猝死增加,QT_c的标准可能变动。

4.4 Frontal Plane QRS Axis

4.4.1 Normal：-30 degrees to +90 degrees

4.4.2 Abnormalities in the QRS Axis：

(1)Left Axis Deviation (LAD)： > -30°(i. e. , lead Ⅱ is mostly "negative")

• Left Anterior Fascicular Block (LAFB)：rS complex (i. e. , small r, big S) in leads Ⅱ, Ⅲ, aVF, small q in leads Ⅰ and /or aVL, and -45° to -90° (see ECG on p14)；in LAFB, the S in lead Ⅲ is > S in lead Ⅱ, and the R in aVL is > R in aVR. This differentiates LAFB from other causes of LAD with rS complexes in Ⅱ, Ⅲ, aVF (e. g. , COPD)

• Some cases of inferior MI with Qr complex in lead Ⅱ (making lead Ⅱ "negative")

• Inferior MI + LAFB in same patient (QS or qrS complex in Ⅱ)

• Some cases of LVH

• Some cases of LBBB

• Ostium primum ASD and other endocardial cushion defects

• Some cases of WPW syndrome (large negative delta wave in lead Ⅱ)

(2)Right Axis Deviation (RAD)： > +90° (i. e. , lead I is mostly "negative")

• Left Posterior Fascicular Block (LPFB)：rS complex in lead Ⅰ, qR in leads Ⅱ, Ⅲ, aVF (however, must first exclude, on clinical basis, causes of right heart overload；these will also give same ECG picture of LPFB)

• Many causes of right heart overload and pulmonary hypertension

• High lateral wall MI with Qr or QS complex in leads Ⅰ and aVL

• Some cases of RBBB

• Some cases of WPW syndrome

• Children, teenagers, and some young adults

(3)Bizarre QRS axis： +150° to -90° (i. e. , lead Ⅰ and lead Ⅱ are both negative)

• Consider limb lead error (usually right and left arm reversal)

• Dextrocardia

• Some cases of complex congenital heart disease

• Some cases of ventricular tachycardia

4.4 额面 QRS 电轴

4.4.1 正常：−30°～+90°

4.4.2 异常的 QRS 电轴

(1)电轴左偏(LAD)：>−30°(如Ⅱ基本为负向波)。

● 左前分支阻滞(LAFB)：Ⅱ，Ⅲ，aVF 呈 rS 型（小 r，大 S），Ⅰ和 aVL 呈 qR 型，电轴 −45°～−90°(见 P15)；SⅢ>SⅡ，R aVL>R Ⅰ，R aVR。LAFB 应和其他原因导致的电轴左偏并伴有Ⅱ、Ⅲ、aVF 呈 rS 型的情况相鉴别[如慢性阻塞性肺部疾病(COPD)]。

● 某些下壁心肌梗死Ⅱ导联呈 Qr 型(Ⅱ以负向波为主)。

● 下壁心肌梗死 +LAFB 同时存在(Ⅱ为 QS 或 qrS)。

● 某些左心室肥厚(LVH)。

● 某些完全性左束支传导阻滞(LBBB)。

● 原发孔未闭型房间隔缺损和其他心内膜垫缺损。

● 某些 WPW 综合征(Ⅱ导联可见大的负向 delta 波)。

(2)电轴右偏(RAD)：>+90°(Ⅰ负向波为主)

● 左后分支阻滞(LPFB)：Ⅰ呈 rS 型，Ⅱ、Ⅲ、aVF 呈 qR 型(必须除外临床右心室超负荷的情况，因为其可以出现与 LPFB 相同的 ECG)。

● 许多引起右心室超负荷和肺高压的因素。

● 高侧壁心肌梗死Ⅰ和 aVL 也可呈 Qr 或 QS 型。

● 某些完全性右束支传导阻滞(RBBB)。

● 某些 WPW 综合征。

● 儿童，青少年，年轻成人。

(3)奇异的 QRS 电轴：+150°到−90°(Ⅰ和Ⅱ都是负向波)

● 考虑导联放置错误(常见左右上肢导联颠倒)。

● 右位心。

● 某些复杂的先天性心脏病。

● 某些室性心动过速。

5 ECG RHYTHM ABNORMALITIES

THINGS TO CONSIDER WHEN ANALYZING ARRHYTHMIAS:

Arrhythmias may be seen on 12-lead ECGs or on rhythm strips of one or more leads. Some arrhythmias are obvious at first glance and don't require intense analysis. Others, however, are more challenging (and often more fun)! They require detective work, i. e., logical thinking. Rhythm analysis is best understood by considering characteristics of impulse formation (if known) as well as impulse conduction. Here are some things to consider as originally conceptualized by Dr. Alan Lindsay (see Fig. 5 – 1):

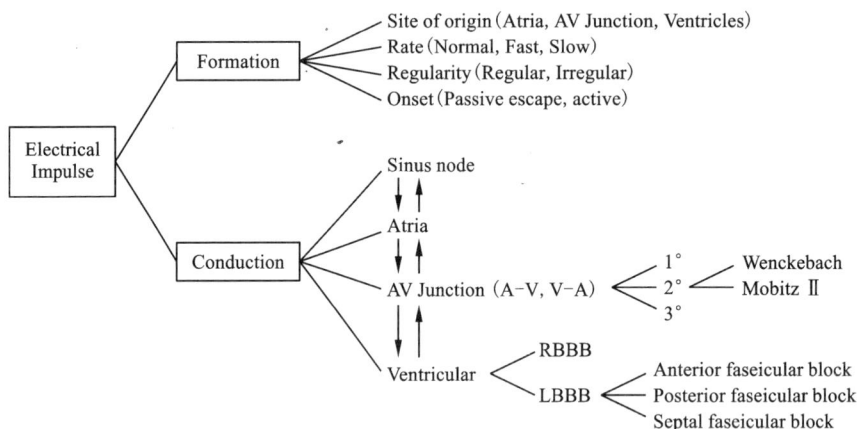

Fig. 5 – 1

(1) Descriptors ofimpulse formation (i. e., the pacemaker or region of impulse formation)

- Site of origin, i. e., where does the rhythm originate?
- Sinus Node (e. g., sinus tachycardia; P waves may be hidden in the preceding T waves at very fast rates)
- Atria (e. g., PACs, ectopic atrial rhythms, etc.)
- AV junction (e. g., PJCs and junctional rhythms)
- Ventricles (e. g., PVCs)
- Rate (i. e., relative to the expected rate for that pacemaker location)
- Accelerated-faster than expected for that pacemaker site (e. g., accelerated junctional rhythms, @ HR = 60 – 100 bpm)
- Slower than expected (e. g., marked sinus bradycardia, 38 bpm)
- Normal (or expected) (e. g., junctional escape rhythm, 45 bpm)

5 心电图节律异常

分析心律失常时应考虑：

心律失常可见于 12 导联心电图或 1 至多个导联。某些心律失常不用费力分析，一眼就可以看出来。而有些则具有挑战性（通常更有趣）！需要探究和逻辑思维。通过思考冲动的形成和传导的特征（如果已知）可以最好地理解节律分析。这就是 Dr. Alan Lindsay 思考问题的初始概念（图 5 − 1）。

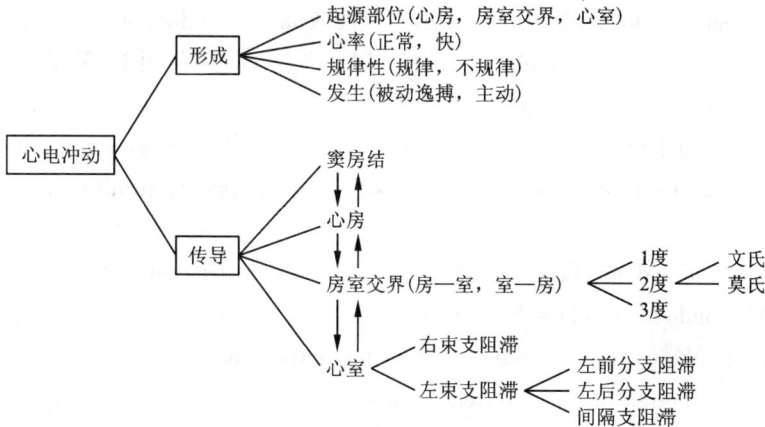

图 5 − 1

（1）冲动形成的描述（如起搏点）

● 起搏部位：该节律源于哪里？

· 窦房结（如窦性心动过速；心率特别快时 P 波可能隐藏在前一个周期的 T 波中）。

· 心房（如房性期前收缩 PACs，异位心房节律等）。

· 房室交界（如交界性期前收缩 PJCs 和交界性心律）。

· 心室（如室性期前收缩 PVCs）。

● 起搏频率（与该部位的预期频率对比）

· 加速并快于该部位的频率（如加速性交界性心律，频率 60 ~ 100 次/min）。

· 慢于预期频率（如明显的窦性心动过缓，38 次/min）。

· 正常（或预期频率）（如交界性逸搏律，45 次/min）。

- Regularity of ventricular and/or atrial response
  - Regular (e. g. , paroxysmal supraventricular tachycardia-PSVT)
  - Regular irregularity (e. g. , ventricular bigeminy)
  - Irregular irregularity (e. g. , atrial fibrillation or MAT)
  - Irregular (e. g. , multifocal PVCs)
- Onset (i. e. , how does arrhythmia begin?)
  - Active onset (e. g. , PAC or PVC, PSVT)
  - Passive onset (e. g. , junctional or ventricular escape beats or rhythms)

(2) Descriptors of impulse conduction (i. e. , how does the abnormal rhythm conduct through the heart chambers?)

- Antegrade (forward) vs. retrograde (backward) conduction
- Conduction delays or blocks: i. e. , 1st, 2nd (type I or II), 3rd degree blocks
- Sites of potential conduction delay
  - Sino-Atrial (SA) block (one can only recognized 2nd degree SA block on the ECG; i. e. , an unexpected failure of a sinus P-wave to appear, resulting in a pause in rhythm)
  - Intra-atrial delay (usually recognized as a widened P wave)
  - AV conduction delays (common)
  - IV blocks (e. g. , bundle branch or fascicular blocks)

Now let's continue with some real rhythms. . .

5.1 Supraventricular Arrhythmias

5.1.1 Premature Atrial Complexes (PAC's)

- Occur as single or repetitive events and have unifocal or multifocal origins.
- The ectopic P wave (often called P′) is often hidden in the ST − T wave of the preceding beat. (Dr. Henry Marriott, master ECG teacher and author, likes to say: "Cherchez le P" which, in French, means: "Search for the P" (on the T wave), and it's clearly sexier to search in French!)
- The P′R interval can be normal or prolonged if the AV junction is partially refractory at the time the premature atrial impulse enters it.
- PAC's can have one of three different outcomes depending on the degree of prematurity (i. e. , coupling interval from previous P wave), and the preceding cycle length (i. e. , RR interval). This is illustrated in Fig. 5 − 2 where normal sinus beats are followed by three possible.

- 心室和/或心房反应的规律性
- 规律（如阵发性室上性心动过速，PSVT）。
- 有规律性的不规律（如室性期前收缩二联律）。
- 无规律性的不规律［如心房纤颤或 MAT（多型房性心动过速）］。
- 不规律（如多源室性期前收缩）。
- 发生（心律失常如何开始的?）
- 主动发生（如房性期前收缩或室性期前收缩，阵发性室上性心动过速等）。
- 被动发生（如交界性或室性逸搏或逸搏心律）。

（2）冲动传导的描述（如异常的节律如何传导到各心腔?）

- 前向传导（向前）与后向传导（向后）。
- 传导延缓或阻滞：如 1 度（1st），2 度（2nd）（type Ⅰ或Ⅱ），3 度（3rd）阻滞。
- 传导延缓的潜在部位
- 窦房阻滞（SAB）（人们在心电图中只能辨认出 2^{nd}度的 SAB；如一个窦性 P 波没有按预期出现，导致节律中出现了一个停顿）。
- 心房内传导延缓（通常通过 P 波增宽来辨认）。
- 房室传导延缓（常见）。
- 心室内传导延缓（如束支或分支阻滞）。

现在让我们来进一步看以下某些真正的节律。

5.1 室上性心律失常

5.1.1 心房性期前收缩（PAC's）

- 可以单个发生或反复出现，可以是单部位或多部位起搏点。
- 异位 P 波（P′）通常隐藏在前一个心搏的 ST－T 中。（Henry Marriott 博士，精通心电图的老师与作者，喜欢说"Cherchez le P"，法语的意思是（在 T 波上）"找 P"，在法语中的含义是非常性感地去寻找的意思!）
- P′R 间期可能正常或延长，当房性期前收缩冲动达到房室结时如果房室结处在部分不应期时，P′R 间期会延长。
- 房性期前收缩（PAC's）可能有三种不同的结局，取决于期前收缩提前的程度（与前一个 P 的配对间期，也称联律间期），以及前一个周期的长短（RR 间期）。图 5－2 描述了正常窦性搏动后分别有 3 个房性期前收缩 PACs（标为 a，b，c，d）的不同命运。

5.1.2 PACs (labeled a, b, c, d in Fig. 5 – 2):

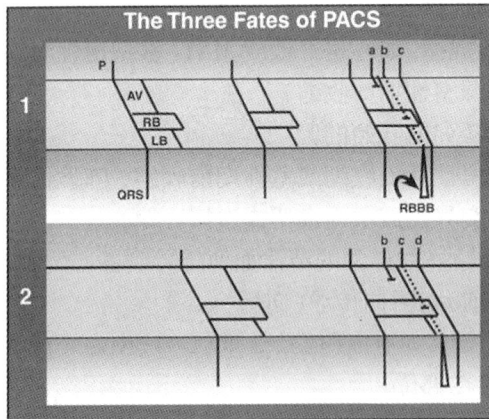

Fig. 5 – 2

● Outcome #1. Nonconducted (or blocked) PAC; i. e. , no QRS complex because the early PAC finds the AV node still refractory to conduction. [see PAC "a" in Fig. 5 – 2 labeled 1, and the nonconducted PAC in ECG shown in Fig. 5 – 3 (arrow); note that it's hidden and slightly distorts the ST – T wave]

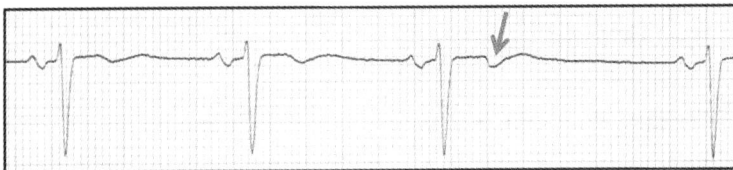

Fig. 5 – 3

● Outcome #2. Conducted with aberration; a PAC conducts to the ventricles but finds one of the 2 bundle branches or one of the LBB fascicles refractory. The resulting QRS is usually wide, and is sometimes called an Ashman beat [see PAC "b" in Fig. 5 – 2, and the V1 rhythm strip in Fig. 5 – 4 showing a PAC with RBBB aberration; note the PAC in the T wave (arrow)].

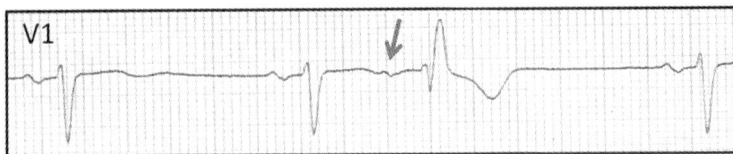

Fig. 5 – 4

● Outcome #3. Normal conduction; i. e. , similar to other QRS complexes in that ECG lead (See PAC "c" and "d" in Fig. 5 – 2).

5.1.2　3个房性期前收缩的不同命运

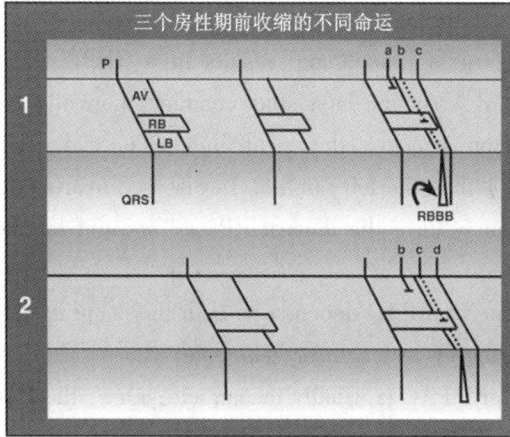

图 5 - 2

● 结果 1. 未下传(或阻滞)的房性期前收缩;未产生 QRS 波群,因为房性期前收缩产生的**太早**,房室结还处在不应期使房性期前收缩不能下传。(见图 5 - 2 的"1"中的 a,而且这个未下传的房性期前收缩如图 5 - 3 心电图中的箭头所示,注意它隐藏在 ST - T 中而且导致 ST - T 有些扭曲或切迹)。

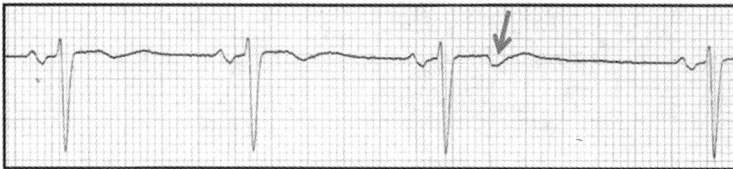

图 5 - 3

● 结果 2. 房性期前收缩伴差异性传导;一个房性期前收缩下传到心室时,左束支或右束支还处在不应期,或者左束支的一个分支不应期还没有过去,这个房性期前收缩后面的 QRS 通常是增宽的,有时被称为阿斯曼(Ashman beat)期前收缩(见图 5 - 2 房性期前收缩 b,图 5 - 4 V1 导联中房性期前收缩伴有右束支传导阻滞型差异性传导;注意房性期前收缩 P'隐藏在 T 波中,如箭头所示)。

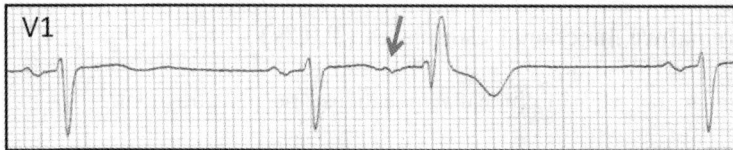

图 5 - 4

● 结果 3. **正常传导**;房性期前收缩下传产生 QRS 波群与该导联中其他 QRS 波群形态一样(见图 5 - 2 中房性期前收缩 c 和 d)。

• In Fig. 5 – 2, labeled "2", the cycle length has increased (slower heart rate). This results in increased refractoriness of all the structures in the conduction system. PAC "b" now can't get through the AV node and isnonconducted; PAC "c" is now blocked in the right bundle branch and results in a RBBB QRS complex (aberrant conduction); PAC "d" occurs later and conducts normally. RBBB aberration is generally more common because the right bundle normally has a slightly longer refractory period (RP) than the left bundle. In diseased hearts either bundle branch or a left bundle fascicle may have the longest RP and account for the aberration in QRS waveform.

Therefore, the fate of a PAC depends on both the coupling interval from the last P wave, and the preceding cycle length or heart rate.

• The pause after a PAC is usually incomplete; i. e. , the PAC actually enters the sinus node and resets its timing, causing the next sinus P to appear earlier than expected (PVCs, on the other hand, are usually followed by a complete pause because the PVC usually does not perturb the sinus node timing; see ECG in Fig. 5 – 5 and Fig. 5 – 18).

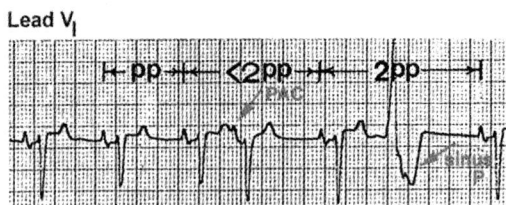

Complete vs Incomplete Pause

Fig. 5 – 5

• "Incomplete" pause：The PP interval surrounding a PAC is less than 2 normal PP intervals (because the PAC reset the sinus timing)

• "Complete" pause：The PP interval surrounding the PVC is equal to 2 normal PP intervals because the sinus continued to fire at its normal rate even though it didn't conduct to the ventricle (see the sinus P hidden in the T wave of the PVC).

5.1.3 Premature Junctional Complexes (PJC's)

• Similar to PAC's in clinical implications, but less frequent.

● 在图 5 - 2 的"2"中,心动周期延长(心率慢),导致了所有的传导系统不应期均延长。房性期前收缩 b 此时不能通过房室结,**未下传**;房性期前收缩 c 阻滞在右束支,导致 QRS 为右束支阻滞图形(**差异性传导**);房性期前收缩"d"发生较晚,传导正常。右束支阻滞图形的差异性传导比较常见,因为右束支的不应期(RP)较左束支略长。但是,心脏在某些病理状态下,左束支或其分支可以有最长的不应期,产生差异性传导的 QRS 可以呈左束支阻滞型。

因此,房性期前收缩的命运取决于:①与前一个 P 波的联律间期;②前一心动周期的长短或心率。

● 房性期前收缩以后的间歇通常是不完全性的;房性期前收缩实际上进入窦房结,重置了时钟,此时的下一个窦性 P 比预期出现的早。但是室性期前收缩(PVC)是完全性的代偿间歇,因为室性期前收缩没有干扰窦房结的时钟(见图 5 - 5 和图 5 - 18)。

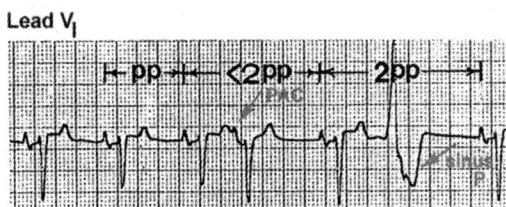

完全性和不完全性间歇

图 5 - 5

● "不完全性"间歇:房性期前收缩(PAC)前后的 PP 间期比 2 个正常的 PP 间期短(因为房性期前收缩重置了窦性时钟)。

● "完全性"间歇:室性期前收缩(PVC)前后的 PP 间期与 2 个正常的 PP 间期相等,因为窦房结继续按自己的正常频率起搏,虽然不能下传到心室[见图 5 - 5,窦性 P 隐藏在室性期前收缩(PVC)的 T 波中]。

5.1.3 交界性期前收缩(PJC's)

● 与房性期前收缩临床意义相似,但较少发生。

● The PJC focus in the AV junction captures the atria (retrograde) and the ventricles (antegrade). The retrograde P wave may appear before, during, or after the QRS complex; if before, the PR interval is usually short (i. e. , <0.12 s). The ECG tracing and ladder diagram shown in Fig. 5 –6 illustrates a classic PJC with retrograde P waves occurring after the QRS.

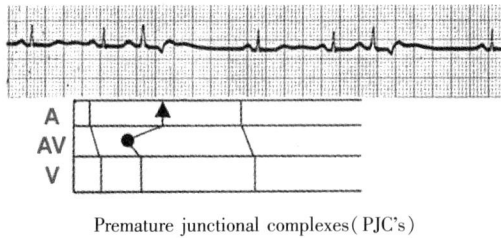

Premature junctional complexes(PJC's)

Fig. 5 –6

5.1.4　Atrial Fibrillation（A-fib）:

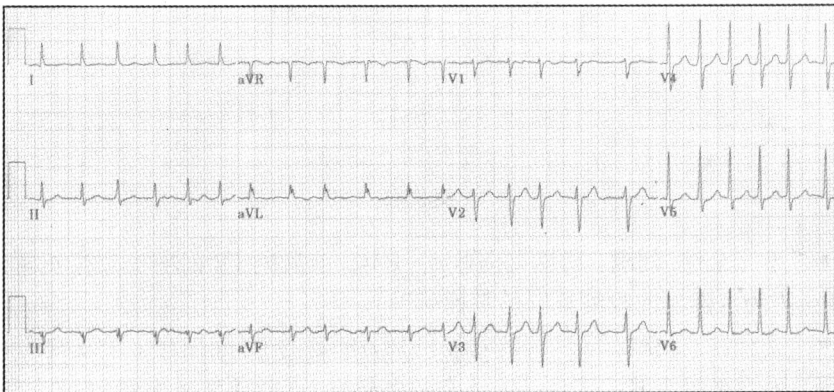

Fig. 5 –7

● Atrial activity is poorly defined; may see course or fine baseline undulations (wiggles) or no atrial activity at all. If atrial activity is seen, it resembles the teeth on an old saw (when compared to atrial flutter that often resembles a new saw or a clean saw-tooth pattern especially in leads Ⅱ, Ⅲ, and aVF).

● Ventricular response (RR intervals) is irregularly irregular and may be fast (HR >100 bpm, indicates inadequate rate control), moderate (HR =60 – 100 bpm), or slow (HR <60 bpm, indicates excessive rate control medication, AV node disease, or drug toxicity such as digoxin). Recent studies indicate that resting HR's <110 bpm may be OK in atrial fibrillation, although not optimal.

● 交界区起搏点发出的冲动既可以逆传夺获心房，也可以前传夺获心室。逆传 P 可以出现在 QRS 的前、中、后，如果出现在 QRS 前 PR 间期通常较短（<0.12 s）。图 5-6 的心电图和梯形图描述了交界性期前收缩的逆传 P 出现在 QRS 之后的典型表现。

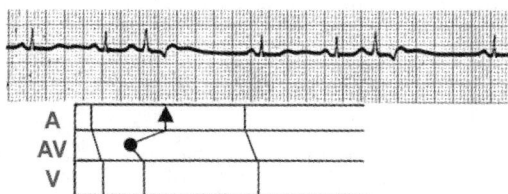

交界性期前收缩（PJC）梯形图（A：心房；AV：房室结；V：心室）

图 5-6

5.1.4 心房纤颤（A-fib）

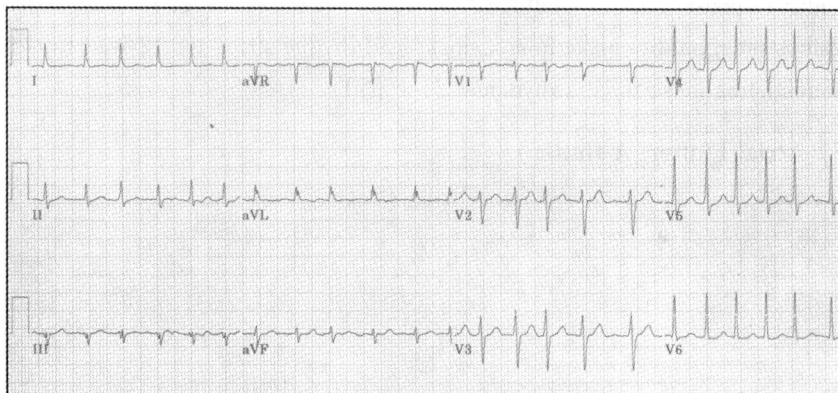

图 5-7

● 很难明确心房活动；可以看到基线起伏（摇摆）或完全见不到心房活动。如果见到心房活动，它像一个旧锯的齿（与心房扑动比较，后者通常像一条新锯，尤其是在 Ⅱ，Ⅲ 和 aVF 导联上完全像一个新锯的锯齿）。

● 心室反应（RR 间期）是无规律性的不规律，可能快（HR > 100 次/min，表明心率控制不当），适度（HR = 60 ~ 100 次/min），或慢（HR < 60 次/min，提示心率过度控制，可能是用药、房室结病变或药物中毒如地高辛所致）。新近研究表明将心房纤颤的静息心率控制到 < 110 次/min 就可以了，尽管不十分理想。

• A regular ventricular response with A-fib usually indicates high grade or complete AV block with an escape or accelerated ectopic pacemaker originating in the AV junction or ventricles (i. e. , consider digoxin toxicity or AV node disease). In the ECG shown in Fig. 5 – 8 the last 2 QRS complexes are junctional escapes indicating high-grade AV block due (note: the last two RR intervals are the same indicating the escape rate).

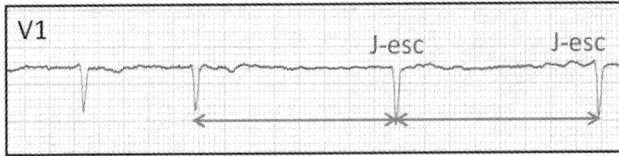

Fig. 5 – 8

• Irregularly-irregular SVT's may also be seen inatrial flutter with an irregular ventricular response and in multifocal atrial tachycardia (MAT). The differential diagnosis is often hard to make from a single lead rhythm strip; the 12-lead ECG is best for differentiating these three arrhythmias (see p50).

5.1.5 Atrial Flutter(A-flutter)

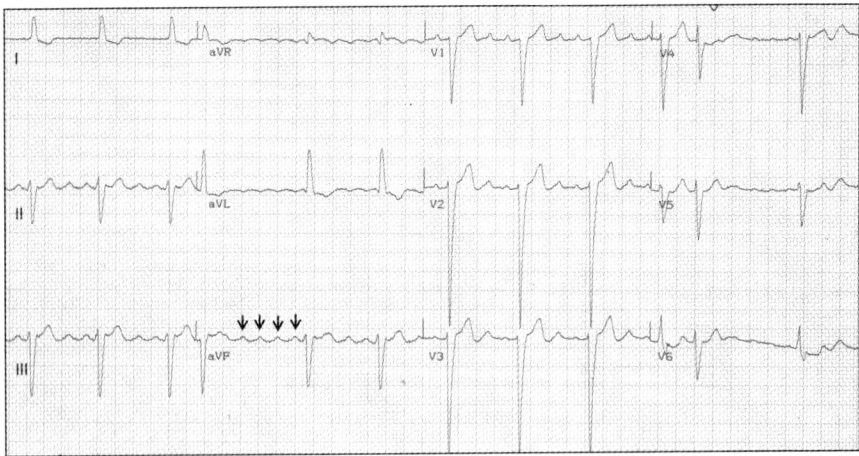

Fig. 5 – 9

• Regular atrial activity usually with a clean saw-tooth appearance in leads Ⅱ, Ⅲ, aVF, and more discrete looking "P" waves in lead V1. The atrial rate is usually about 300/min, but may be as slow as 150 – 200/min or as fast as 400 – 450/min. The above ECG also shows LVH and left anterior fascicular block (LAFB).

● 如果心房纤颤时心室反应很**规律**通常提示有**高度的或完全性的房室传导阻滞**,伴有交界性或心室逸搏,或加速性的交界区或心室的异位起搏心律(如地高辛中毒或房室结病变)。图 5-8 心电图显示的最后 2 个 QRS 波就是交界性逸搏,提示高度的房室阻滞(注意:最后 2 个 RR 间期相等提示逸搏频率)。RR 之间的小 f 波均未能下传心室,直到房室结逸搏按房室结周期开始逸搏。

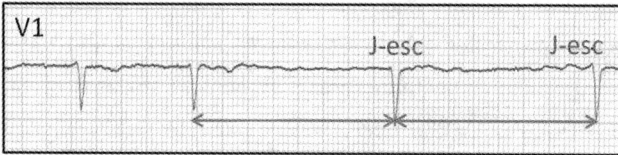

图 5-8

● **无规律性的不规律室上性心动过速**也可以见于**心房扑动**伴有一个不规律的心室反应以及**多源性房性心动过速(MAT)**。从单一的导联中很难作出鉴别诊断,12 导联心电图对于鉴别这 3 种心律失常更好(见 P51)。

5.1.5 心房扑动(A-flutter)

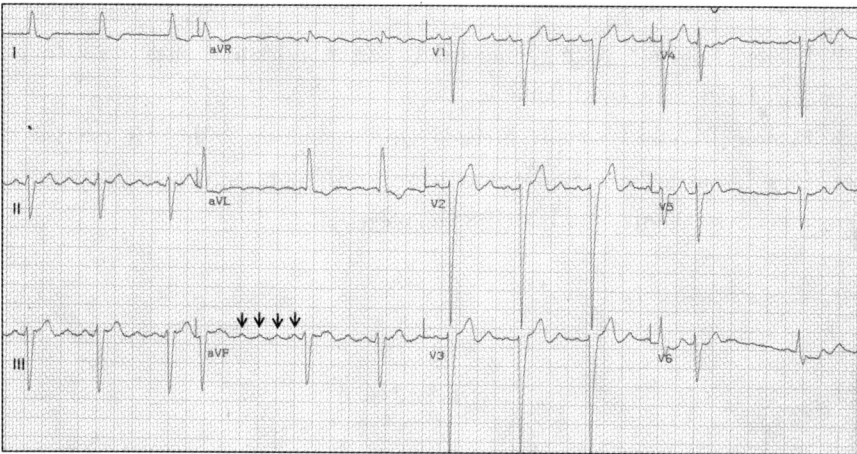

图 5-9

● 有规律的心房扑动通常可以在Ⅱ,Ⅲ,aVF 导联上表现为清晰的锯齿样图形,V1 导联可见更多的离散的"P"波(F 波)。心房率通常 300 次/min,但也可以慢到 150~200 次/min 或快达 400~450 次/min. 上面的心电图同时存在左心室肥厚(LVH)和左前分支阻滞(LAFB)。

• Untreated A-flutter often presents with a 2∶1 A-V conduction ratio. This a commonly missed arrhythmia diagnosis because the flutter waves are often difficult to find. Therefore, always think "atrial flutter with 2∶1 block" whenever there is a regular SVT @ approximately 150 bpm! (You aren't likely to miss it if you look for it.). In the 12-lead ECG shown above both 2∶1 and 4∶1 ratios are seen.

• The ventricular response may be 2∶1, 3∶1 (rare), 4∶1, or variable depending upon AV conduction properties. A-flutter with 2∶1 block is illustrated in the rhythm strip in Fig. 5 – 10; one of the flutter waves occurs at the end of the QRS (pseudo RBBB pattern). Atrial rate ＝280 bpm, ventricular rate ＝140 bpm.

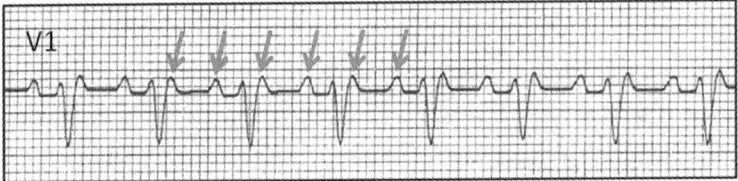

Fig. 5 – 10

5.1.6 Ectopic Atrial Tachycardia and Rhythms

• Ectopic, discrete looking, unifocal P′ waves with atrial rates ＜250/min (not to be confused with slow atrial flutter).

• Ectopic P′ waves usually precede QRS complexes with P′R interval ＜ RP′ interval (i. e. , not to be confused with paroxysmal supraventricular tachycardia with retrograde P waves shortly after the QRS complexes).

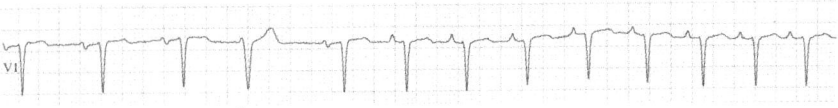

Fig. 5 – 11

• The ECG in Fig. 5 – 11 shows 3 beats of sinus rhythm, a PVC, a sinus beat, and the onset of an ectopic atrial tachycardia (note the different P wave morphology)

• Ventricular response may be 1∶1 (as ECG in Fig. 5 – 11) or with varying degrees of AV block (especially in the setting of digitalis toxicity).

• Ectopic atrial rhythms are similar to ectopic atrial tachycardia, but with HR ＜ 100 bpm. The ectopic "P" wave morphology is clearly different from the sinus P wave.

● 未治疗的心房扑动通常表现为 2:1 的房室传导。这常常导致心律失常的诊断被漏掉，因为通常很难发现心房扑动波。因此，无论何时遇到一个**有规律的室上性心动过速**时，如果频率在 **150 次/min**，一定要想到可能是"**心房扑动伴 2:1 阻滞**"(如果你想到了就不会漏掉)。在 12 - 导联心电图上也可以看到 2:1 和 4:1 的传导比例。

● 心室反应可能是 2:1，3:1(偶见)，4:1，或根据房室传导的性能而变化。图 5 - 10 是一例伴有 2:1 传导阻滞的心房扑动，其中 1 个心房扑动波与 QRS 末端融合(假的右束支传导阻滞)。心房率 = 280 次/min，心室率 = 140 次/min。

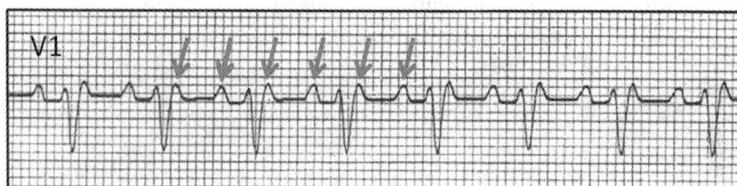

图 5 - 10

5.1.6 异位房性心动过速和心房律

● 看上去离散的，单源的异位 P' 波，心房率 < 250 次/min，一般不会和慢性心房扑动相混淆。

● 异位 P' 波通常出现在 QRS 前而且 P'R 间期 < RP' 间期(因此可以和阵发性室上性心动过速相鉴别，后者的逆传 P 可出现在 QRS 后而且 RP' 很短)。

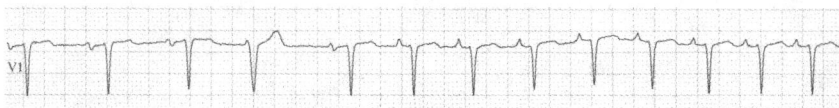

图 5 - 11

● 图 5 - 11 的心电图中有 3 个是窦性心律，1 个室性期前收缩，1 个窦性波，之后发生了一串异位房性心动过速(注意 P 波形态不同)。

● 心室反应 1:1(见图 5 - 11)而且伴有不同程度的房室传导阻滞(特别是处于地高辛中毒时)。

● 异位心房律与异位房性心动过速相似，但 HR < 100 次/min，异位"P"波的形态与窦性 P 波形态明显不同。

5.1.7 Multifocal Atrial Tachycardia (MAT) and rhythm

• Discrete, multifocal P′ waves occurring at rates of 100 – 250/min and with varying P′R intervals (one should see at least 3 different P waves morphologies in a given lead).

• Ventricular response is irregularly irregular (i. e. , often confused with A-fib).

• May be intermittent, alternating with periods of normal sinus rhythm.

• Seen most often in elderly patients with chronic or acute medical problems such as exacerbation of chronic obstructive pulmonary disease.

• If atrial rate is < 100 bpm, call it multifocal atrial rhythm.

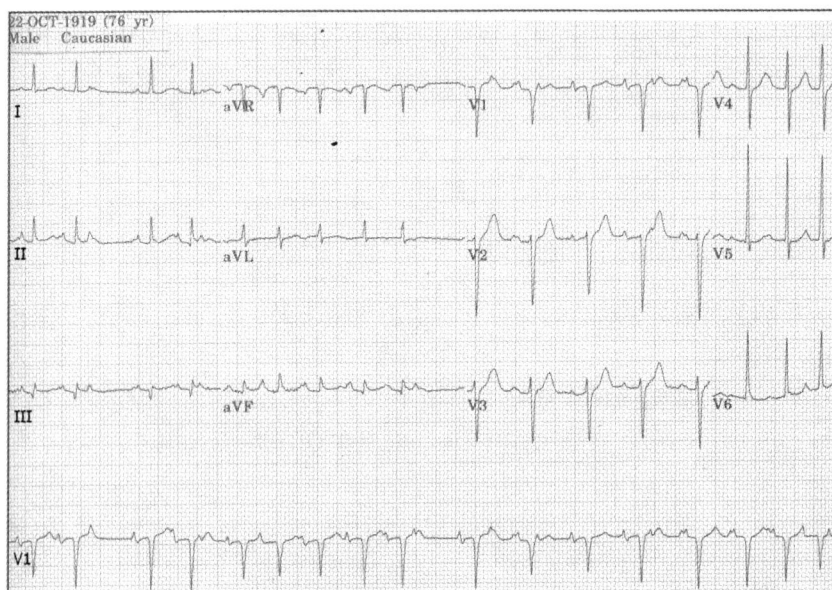

Fig. 5 – 12

Look at lead V1 for the discrete multifocal P waves of MAT, and how other leads look just like a-fibrillation (e. g. , leads aVL and V4)

5.1.8 Paroxysmal Supraventricular Tachycardia(PSVT)

Basic Considerations: These arrhythmias are circus movement tachycardias that use the mechanism of reentry; they are also called reciprocating tachycardias. The onset is sudden, usually initiated by a premature beat, and the arrhythmia stops abruptly-which is why they are called paroxysmal tachycardias. They are usually narrow-QRS tachycardias unless there is preexisting bundle branch block (BBB) or aberrant ventricular conduction (i. e. , rate related BBB). There are several types of PSVT depending on the location of the reentry circuit. The diagram in Fig. 5 – 13 illustrates the mechanism for AV nodal reentrant tachycardia, the most common form of PSVT.

5.1.7 多源房性心动过速(MAT)和心房律

* 离散的,多源的 P'波频率在 100~250 次/min 而且伴有 P'R 间期的变化(在一个导联中可以见到至少 3 种形态的 P 波)。
* 心室反应为无规律的不规律(通常与心房纤颤相混淆)。
* 可以是一过性的或者与正常窦性心律交替出现。
* 常见于伴有慢性或急性临床问题的老年患者,如恶化的慢性阻塞性肺疾病。
* 如果心房率 <100 次/min,称作多源性房性心律。

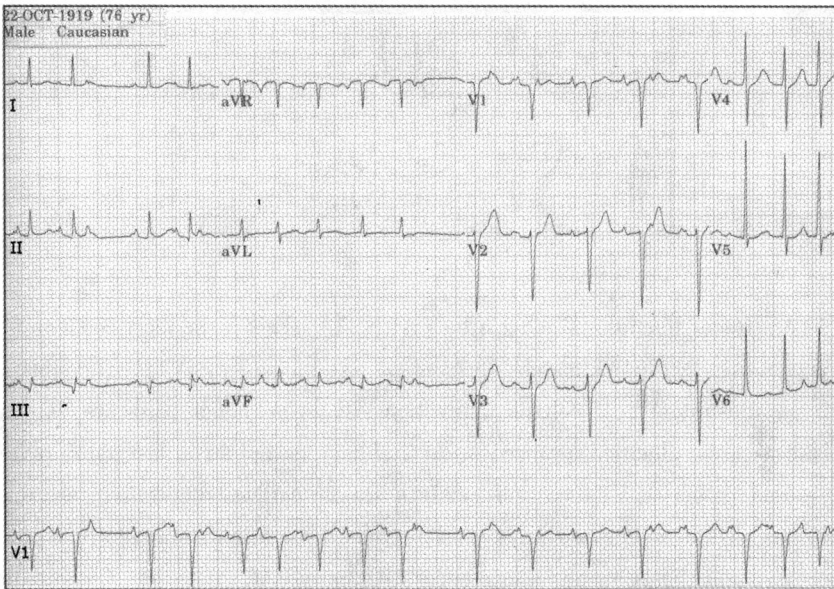

图 5-12

看 V1 导联是多源性房性心动过速的离散的多源的 P 波,而其他导联看上去就像心房纤颤(如 aVL 和 V4)。

5.1.8 阵发性室上性心动过速(PSVT)

基本解读: 这些心律失常是**折返型心动过速**,其发生机制是折返。也称为**往返运动型心动过速**。通常是突然发生,由一个期前收缩诱发,而且这个心律失常可以突然中断,因此称之为阵发性心动过速。它们通常是窄 QRS 心动过速,除非以前就有束支阻滞(BBB)或心室的差异性传导(如频率相关性 BBB)。发生折返的部位不同,阵发性室上性心动过速的类型也不同。图 5-13 描述了**房室结折返性心动过速**的发生机制,也是最常见的室上性心动过速。

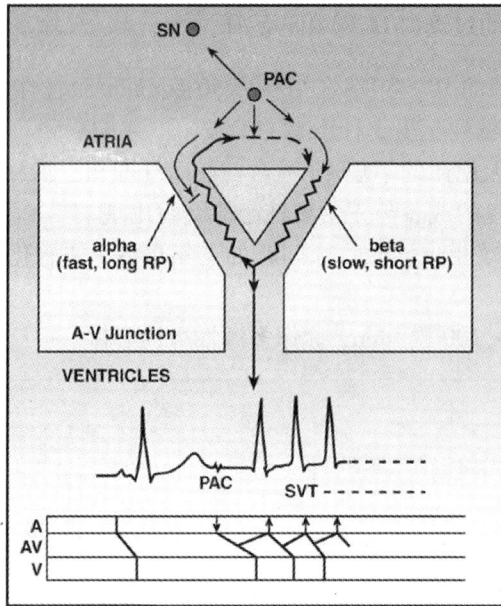

Fig. 5 – 13

(1) AV Nodal Reentrant Tachycardia (AVNRT) : This is the most common form of PSVT accounting for approximately 75% of all symptomatic PSVTs. The diagram in Fig. 5 – 13 illustrates the mechanism involving dual AV nodal pathways, alpha and beta, with different electrical properties. In the diagram alpha is a fast pathway but has a long refractory period (RP), and betais a slower pathway but with a shorter RP. During sinus rhythm alpha is always used because it is faster, and there is plenty of time between sinus beats for alpha to recover. An early PAC, however, finds alpha still refractory and enters the slower beta pathway to reach the ventricles. As it slowly traverses beta, however, alpha recovers allowing retrograde conduction back to the atria. The retrograde P wave (sometimes called an atrial echo) is often simultaneous with or just after the QRS and not easily seen on the ECG, but it can reenter the AV junction because of beta's short RP and continue the tachycardia.

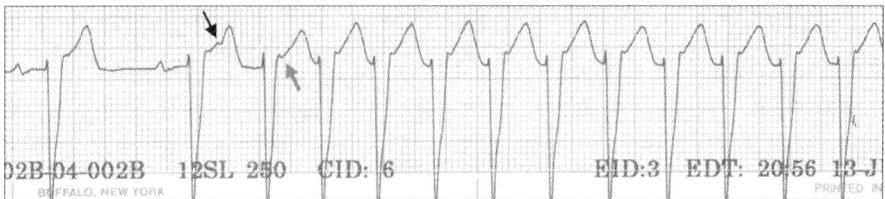

Fig. 5 – 14

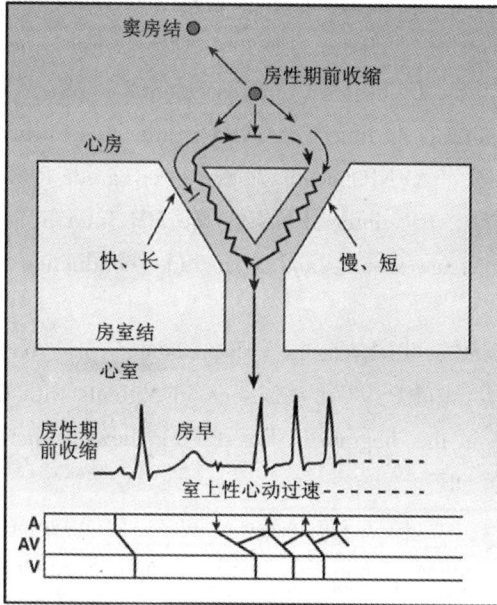

图 5 - 13

（1）房室结折返型心动过速（AVNRT）：**这是最常见的室上性心动过速，大约占症状型阵发性室上性心动过速的75%**。图 5 - 13 描述的发生机制主要是房室结双通道，**alpha** 和 **beta** 通道各自具有不同的电特性。**alpha** 通道是快通道但是不应期长，而 **beta** 是慢通道而不应期短。正常窦性心律总是通过 **alpha** 快通道下传，因为传导快，而且 2 个窦性冲动之间有足够的时间去恢复 **alpha** 通道的不应期。但是当一个房性期前收缩下传到房室结时发现 **alpha** 依然在不应期，只好进入慢通道 **beta**（不应期短，已结束）到达心室。由于在通过 **beta** 慢通道时速度较慢，**alpha** 不应期结束并可以允许电活动逆传到心房。这个逆传 P（有时称为**心房回声**）几乎同时与 QRS 产生，或刚好在 QRS 之后，所以在 ECG 上很难发现，但是它能在房室结内形成折返，使心动过速持续下去。

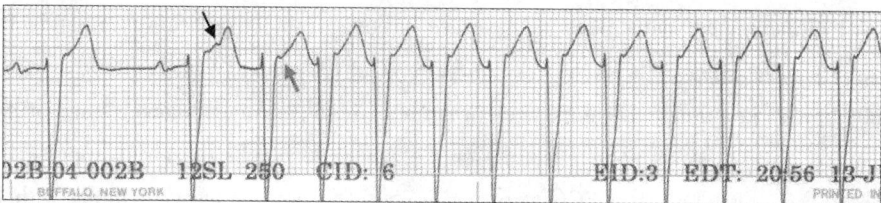

图 5 - 14

In the ECG shown in Fig. 5 – 14 2 sinus beats are followed by PAC (first arrow) that initiates the onset of PSVT. Retrograde P waves (second arrow) immediately follow each QRS (seen as a little dip at onset of ST segment).

If an early PAC is properly timed, AVNRT results as seen in the diagram on p54. Rarely, an atypical form of AVNRT occurs with the retrograde P wave appearing in front of the next QRS (i. e. , RP′ interval > 1/2 the RR interval), implying antegrade conduction down the faster alpha, and retrograde conduction up the slower beta pathway.

(2) AV Reciprocating Tachycardia (Extranodal bypass pathway): This is the second most common form of PSVT and is seen in patients with the WPW syndrome. The WPW ECG, seen in the diagram in Fig. 4 – 1, shows a short PR, a delta wave, and somewhat widened QRS.

This type of PSVT can also occur in the absence of the typical WPW pattern if the accessory pathway only allows conduction in the retrograde direction (i. e. , concealed WPW). Like AVNRT, the onset of PSVT is usually initiated by a PAC that finds the bypass track temporarily refractory, conducts down the slower AV junction into the ventricles, and reenters the atria through the bypass track. In this type of PSVT retrograde P waves usually appear shortly after the QRS in the ST segment (i. e. , RP′ <1/2 RR interval). Rarely the antegrade limb for this PSVT uses the bypass track, and the retrograde limb uses the AV junction; the PSVT then resembles a wide QRS tachycardia and must be differentiated from ventricular tachycardia.

(3) Sino-Atrial Reentrant Tachycardia: This is a rare form of PSVT where the reentrant circuit is between the sinus node and the right atria. The ECG looks just like sinus tachycardia, but the tachycardia is paroxysmal; i. e. , it starts and ends abruptly.

5.1.9 Junctional Rhythms and Tachycardias

(1) Junctional Escape Beats: These are passive, protective beats originating from subsidiary pacemaker cells in the AV junction. The pacemaker's basic firing rate is 40 – 60 bpm; junctional escapes are programmed to occur whenever the primary pacemaker (i. e. , sinus node) defaults or the AV node blocks the atrial impulse from reaching the ventricles. The ECG strip in Fig. 5 – 15 shows sinus arrhythmia with two junctional escapes (arrows). Incomplete AV dissociation is also seen during the junctional escapes.

图 5 - 14 的心电图中，2 个窦性搏动后跟随一个房性期前收缩（第一个箭头所示），它触发了阵发性室上性心动过速的发生。每个 QRS 波后紧随一个逆传 P 波（第二个箭头），在 ST 段的起始部形成一个小的向下的切迹。

如果一个房性期前收缩在时间上提前的恰到好处，就可以见到 P55 中所示的房室结折返型心动过速。极为少见的情况下，一个典型的房室结折返型心动过速的逆传 P 波出现在下一个 QRS 的前面（如 RP′间期 >1/2RR 间期），意味着前传通过 **alpha** 快通道，而逆传通过 **beta** 慢通道。

（2）房室折返型心动过速（房室结外旁路）：这是排在第二常见的阵发性室上性心动过速，见于预激综合征（WPW syndrome）。见图 4 - 1 的 ECG，可见短的 PR，1 个 delta 波和宽大的 QRS 波。

这种类型的阵发性室上性心动过速也可以看不到上述典型的 WPW 特征，因为有的旁路只能逆传（如隐匿性预激）。和房室结折返型心动过速一样，房室折返型心动过速通常也是由一个房性期前收缩引起，房性期前收缩下传时，旁路临时处在不应期，只好沿着房室结缓慢下传到心室，然后从旁路（不应期已过）逆传回到心房。这种类型的室上性心动过速的逆传 P 出现在 ST 段紧随 QRS 之后（RP′< 1/2 RR 间期）。少数情况下，阵发性室上性心动过速前传通过旁路（kent 束）而逆传通过房室结；这样的阵发性室上性心动过速很像宽 QRS 室性心动过速，而且必须与室性心动过速相鉴别。

（3）窦房折返型心动过速：在阵发性室上性心动过速中比较少见，折返环在窦房结和右心房之间。ECG 看上去像窦性心动过速，而且是阵发性的，突然发生和突然停止。

5.1.9 交界性心律和心动过速

（1）交界性逸搏：是来自于房室结辅助起搏细胞的被动的保护性的搏动。起搏基本频率为 40~60 次/min；当原始起搏点（窦房结）违约时，或房室结阻滞了心房冲动使其不能传到心室时，交界性逸搏按自己的程序出现。图 5 - 15 的 ECG 显示窦性心律失常伴有 2 个交界性逸搏（箭头），并可以看到不完全的房室分离。

（2）Junctional Escape Rhythm：This is a sequence of 3 or more junctional escape beatsoccurring by default at a rate of 40 – 60 bpm. There may be AV dissociation, or the atria can be captured retrogradely from the junctional focus.

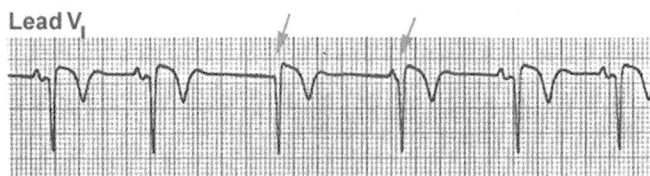

Incomplete AV dissociation due to sinus slowing（default）
with junctional escapes（arrows）

Fig. 5 – 15

（3）Accelerated Junctional Rhythm：This is an active junctional pacemaker rhythm caused by events that perturb the pacemaker cells in the AV junction（e. g. , ischemia, drugs, and electrolyte abnormalities）. The rate is 60 – 100 bpm）.

（4）Nonparoxysmal Junctional Tachycardia：This usually begins as an accelerated junctional rhythm but the heart rate gradually increases to > 100 bpm. There may be AV dissociation, or retrograde atrial capture may occur. Ischemia（usually from right coronary artery occlusion in inferior MI patients）and digitalis intoxication are the two most common causes.

5.2 Ventricular Arrhythmias

5.2.1 Premature Ventricular Complexes（PVCs）

PVCs may beunifocal, multifocal or multiformed. Multifocal PVCs have different sites of origin, which means their coupling intervals（from previous QRS complexes）are usually different. Multiformed PVCs usually have the same coupling intervals （because they originate in the same ectopic site but their conduction through the ventricles differs. Multiformed PVCs are common in digitalis intoxication. PVCs occur as isolated single events or as couplets, triplets, and salvos（4 – 6 PVCs in a row）also called brief ventricular tachycardias.

In Fig. 5 – 16 " A " illustrates single PVCs and PVC couplets; " B " illustrates interpolated PVCs（sandwiched between 2 sinus beats；the PR after the PVC is prolonged because the PVC retrogradely entered the AV junction）; " C " illustrates end-diastolic PVCs with and w/o fusion.

（2）交界性逸搏心律：窦房结违约时如出现 3 个或 3 个以上的连续的交界性逸搏称之为**交界性心律**，频率在 **40 ~ 60 次/min**。可以有房室分离，或交界区的逆传夺获心房。

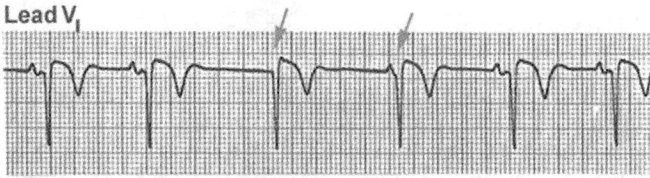

由于窦缓（窦房结违约）引起的房室分离伴有交界性逸搏（箭头所示）

图 5 - 15

（3）加速性交界性自主节律（或加速性交界性心律）：这是一种交界区主动起搏的节律，频率为 60 ~ 100 次/min。通常因为缺血、药物和电解质紊乱等干扰了房室结的起搏细胞所致。

（4）非阵发性交界性心动过速：通常始于加速性交界性自主节律，但是心率逐渐增加到 > 100 次/min，可能有房室分离，或逆传夺获心房。心肌缺血（常见于下壁心肌梗死，右冠状动脉堵塞）和地高辛中毒是两种最常见的原因。

5.2 室性心律失常

5.2.1 室性期前收缩（PVCs）

PVCs 可以是单源的，多源的或多型的。多源 PVCs 有多个不同的起搏点，这就意味着它们的配对间期（联律间期，从前面的正常的 QRS 起始部到期前收缩的 QRS′的起始部）常常不同。多形性 PVCs 通常有相同的配对间期，因为它们源于相同的异位起搏点，但是它们因在心室内的传导不同而产生不同形态的 QRS′，多形性 PVCs 常见于地高辛中毒。PVCs 是单一的孤立事件，成对室性期前收缩、3 个或 4 ~ 6 个连续出现成一排的也称短阵室性心动过速。

图 5 - 16A 是单发 **PVCs** 和成对的 **PVCs**；B 是**间位 PVCs**（像三明治一样夹在 2 个窦性波之间，**PVC** 后面的 PR 是延长的，异位 PVC 逆传进入了房室结）；C 是舒张晚期室性期前收缩 **PVCs** 伴或不伴室性融合波。

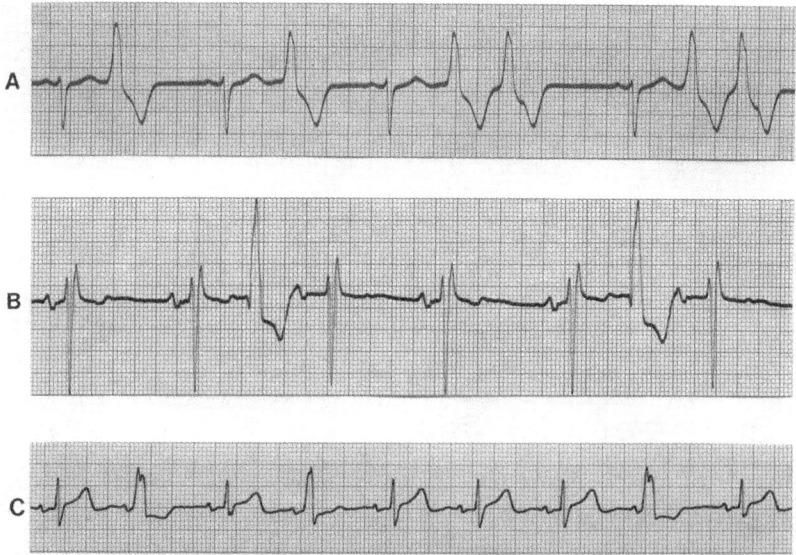

Fig. 5－16

PVCs may occur early in the cycle (R-on-T phenomenon), after the T wave, or late in the cycle-often fusing with the next QRS (called a fusion beat; see 2nd PVC in "C"). R-on-T PVCs may be especially dangerous in acute ischemic settings, because the ventricles are more vulnerable to ventricular tachycardia or fibrillation. In the example below, late (end-diastolic) PVCs are illustrated with varying degrees of fusion. For fusion to occur the sinus P wave must have made it into the ventricles to start the ventricular activation sequence. Before ventricular activation is completed, however, the "late" PVC occurs, and the resultant QRS looks a bit like the normal QRS, and a bit like the PVC; i. e., a fusion QRS (see arrows). Also, see the second PVC with fusion in "C".

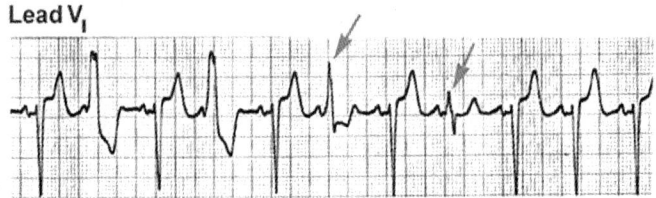

Parasystolic PVC's with fusions (arrows)

Fig. 5－17

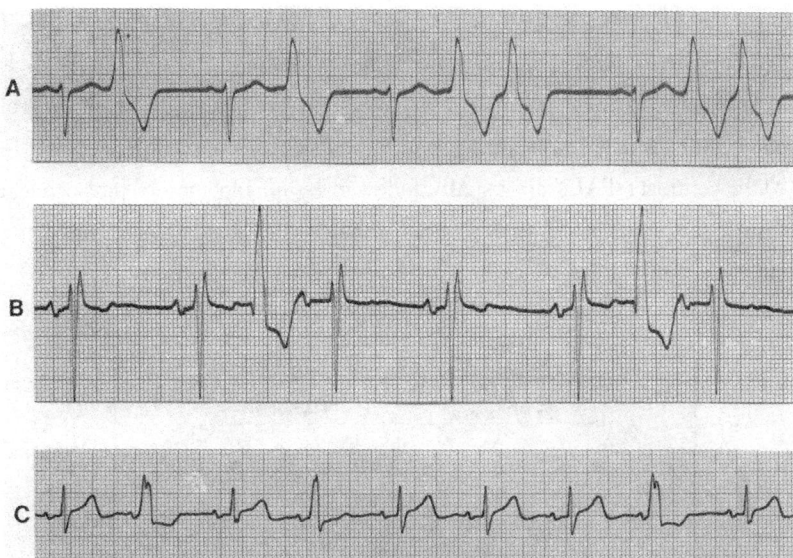

图 5－16

　　PVCs 可以在周期中发生较早(R－on－T 现象),可出现在 T 波之后或周期之末,常与下一个 QRS 融合(叫室性融合波;见图 5－16C 的第 2 和第 3 个 PVC),R－on－T PVCs 尤其重要,在急性缺血的情况下容易诱发室性心动过速和室颤。在下面的例子中,舒张晚期室性期前收缩有不同程度的融合。融合的先决条件是窦性 P 波一定要进入心室并按顺序开始兴奋心室,然而在心室兴奋还没有完成时,"迟到"的室性期前收缩来到了,并兴奋了还没有兴奋的部分心室,所以这个合成的 QRS 看起来有点像正常的 QRS,还有点像 PVC,例如 1 个融合的 QRS(见箭头)。见图 5－16C 中的第二个 PVC。

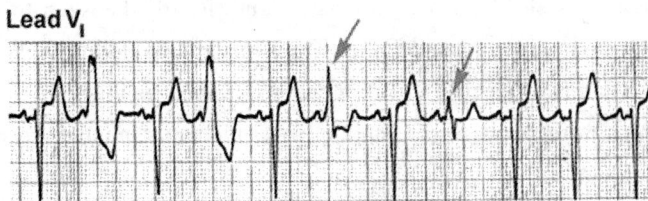

并行性室性期前收缩伴融合波(箭头)

图 5－17

The events following a PVC are of interest. Usually a PVC is followed by a complete compensatory pause, because the sinus node timing is not interrupted by the PVC; one sinus P wave near the PVC can't reach the ventricles because the ventricles are refractory after the PVC; the next sinus P wave occurs on time based on the basic sinus rate. In contrast, PACs are usually followed by an incomplete pause because the PAC can reset the sinus node timing; this enables the next sinus P wave to appear earlier than expected. These concepts are illustrated in the diagram below.

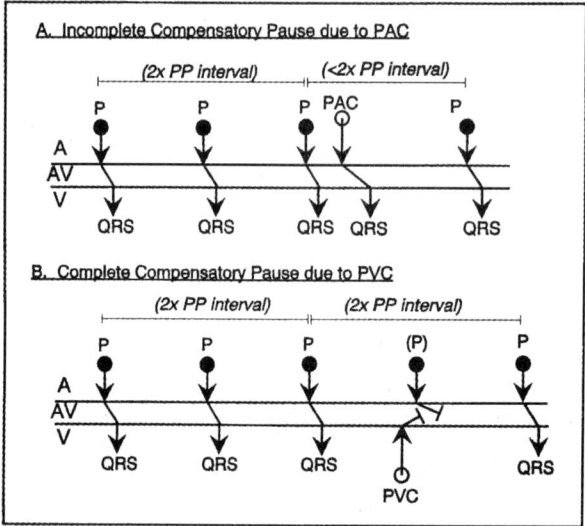

Fig. 5 – 18

Not all PVCs are followed by a pause. If a PVC occurs early enough (especially when the sinus rate is slow), it may appear "sandwiched" between two normal sinus beats. This is called aninterpolated PVC. The sinus P wave following the PVC usually has a longer PR interval because of retrograde concealed conduction by the PVC into the AV junction slowing subsequent conduction of the sinus impulse (see "B" in Fig. 5 – 16).

Rarely a PVC may retrogradely capture the atrium and reset the sinus node timing resulting in an incomplete pause. Often the retrograde P wave can be seen on the ECG, hiding in the ST – T wave of the PVC.

跟随 PVC 后面的情况也很有意思。PVC 通常跟随一个完全性代偿间歇，因为窦房结时钟没有被 PVC 干扰；距 PVC 较近的窦性 P 波不能达到心室，因为心室正处在室性期前收缩后的不应期；下一个窦性 P 波根据窦性频率按时产生。相比之下，房性期前收缩（PACs）通常跟随一个不完全代偿间歇，因为 PAC 能够重置窦房结的时钟；导致下一个窦性 P 波比预期的要提前出现。图 5 - 18 描述了这个概念。

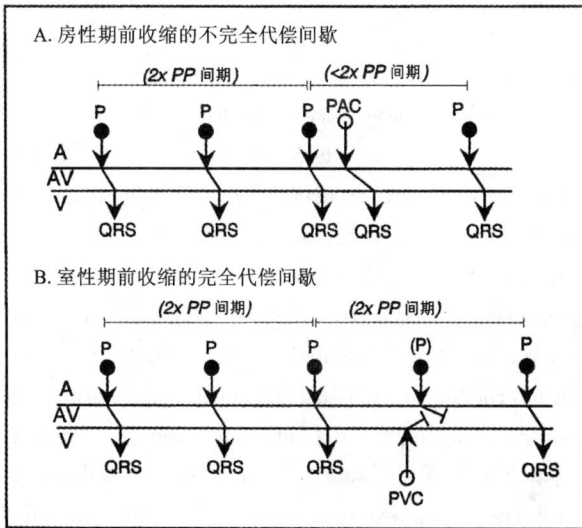

图 5 - 18

并不是所有的 PVC 都有间歇，如果 PVC 出现的足够早（尤其是当窦性频率比较慢的时候），它可以"像三明治"一样出现在 2 个正常窦性波动中间，叫**间位室性期前收缩**。PVC 后面的窦性 P 波通常 PR 间期较长，因为 PVC 产生的进入房室结的隐匿传导减慢了窦性冲动的顺序传导（见图 5 - 16B）。

很少有 PVC 可以逆传并夺获心房，并且重置窦房结的时钟产生一个不完全代偿间歇。ECG 通常可以见到逆传 P，常常隐藏在 PVC 产生的 ST - T 中。

Lead V$_1$

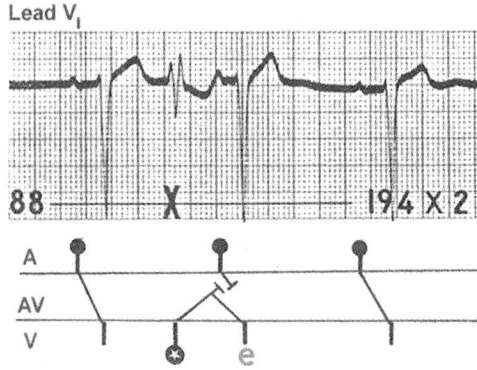

Interpolated PVC with ventricular echo (e)

Fig. 5 − 19

A most unusual post-PVC event occurs when retrograde activation of the AV junction (or atria) re-enters (or comes back to) the ventricles as a ventricular echo. This is illustrated in Fig. 5 − 19. The "ladder" diagram under the ECG helps us understand the mechanism. The P wave following the PVC is the sinus P wave, but the PR interval is too short for it to have caused the next QRS. (Remember, the PR interval following an interpolated PVC is usually longer than normal, not shorter!). The PVC reenters the ventricles within the AV junction. Amazing, isn't it?

PVCs usually stick out like "sore thumbs" or funny-looking-beats (FLB's), because they are bizarre in appearance compared to the normal QRS complexes. However, not all premature "sore thumbs" are PVCs. In the example in Fig. 5 − 20 2 PACs are seen: #1 has a normal QRS, and #2 has RBBB aberrancy-which looks like a sore thumb. The challenge, therefore, is to recognize sore thumbs for what they are, and that's the next topic for discussion!

Not all sore thumbs are PVC's

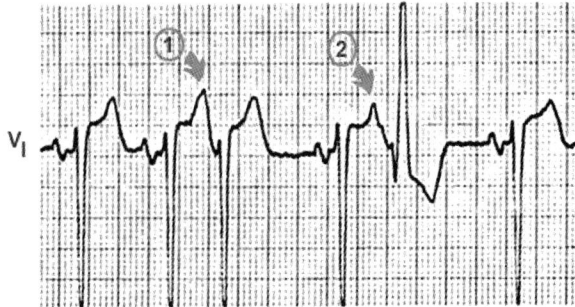

PAC(1) with normal IV conduction

PAC(2) with RBBB aberration (note: longer preceding cycle prior to aberrancy)

Fig. 5 −20

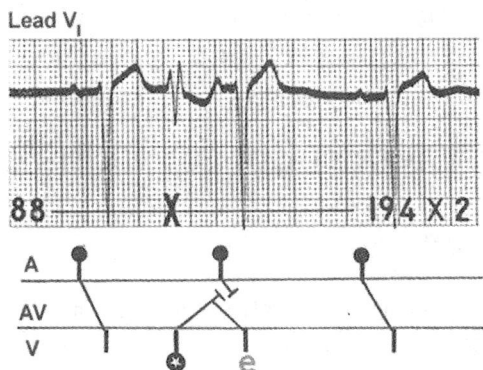

插入性室性期前收缩伴心室回声

图 5 – 19

还有一种非常少见的室性期前收缩后事件。当逆传兴奋了房室结或心房后返回到心室,称**心室回声**。图 5 – 19 中的梯形图有助于我们理解其产生机制。PVC后面的 P 波是窦性 P 波,但是 PR 间期太短以至于不能认为是它产生的后面的QRS(注意,间位 PVC 后面的 PR 间期应该较正常 PR 长,绝不会短!)。这个 PVC从房室结又回到心室。真是令人惊讶!

PVCs 通常显得"令人瞩目"或滑稽波形(FLB's),因为看上去比正常的 QRS波显得奇怪。但是,并不是所有的"令人瞩目"波都是室性期前收缩(PVCs)。图 5–20 是 2 个 PACs 的例子:图中①房性期前收缩的 QRS 正常,而图中②房性期前收缩产生了右束支阻滞差异性传导——看起来"令人瞩目"。因此,如何识别这个到底是房性期前收缩还是室性期前收缩是一个挑战!这就是接下来要讨论的话题。注意图 5 – 20 中②房性期前收缩之所有产生差异性传导是因为它前面有一个较长的周期。

并不是所有"令人瞩目"的波都是室性期前收缩

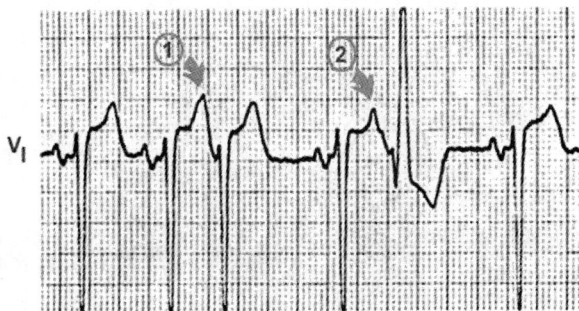

PAC(1):QRS 正常

PAC(2):产生了右束支传导阻滞差异性传导

图 5 – 20

（The following section on "Aberrant Ventricular Conduction" was written jointly by Drs. Alan Lindsay, Frank Yanowitz, and J. Douglas Ridges in the 1980's. Slight modifications from the original have been made. ）

5.3 ABERRENT VENTRICULAR CONDUCTION

5.3.1 INTRODUCTION

Aberrant ventricular conduction（AVC）is a very common source of confusion in interpreting 12-lead ECGs and rhythm strips. A thorough understanding of its mechanism and recognition is essential to all persons who read ECGs.

Before we can understand aberrant ventricular conduction we must first review how normal conduction of the electrical impulse occurs in the heart（Fig. 5 – 21）. What a magnificent design! Impulses from the fastest center of automaticity（SA node）are transmitted through the atria and over specialized fibers（Bachmann's bundle to the left atrium and three internodal tracts）to the AV node. The AV node provides sufficient conduction delay to allow atrial contraction to contribute to ventricular filling. Following slow AV node conduction high velocity conduction tracts deliver the electrical impulse to the right and left ventricles（through the His bundle, bundle branches and fascicles, and into he Purkinje network）. Simultaneous activation of the two ventricles results in a NARROW, NORMAL QRS COMPEX（0. 06 – 0. 1 sec QRS duration）. Should conduction delay or block in one of the bundle branches occur then an ABNORMAL WIDE QRS COMPLEX will result. （A delay or block in a fascicle of the left bundle branch will also result in an abnormal QRS that is not necessarily wide but of a different shape（i. e. , a change in frontal plane QRS axis）from the person's normal QRS morphology. ）

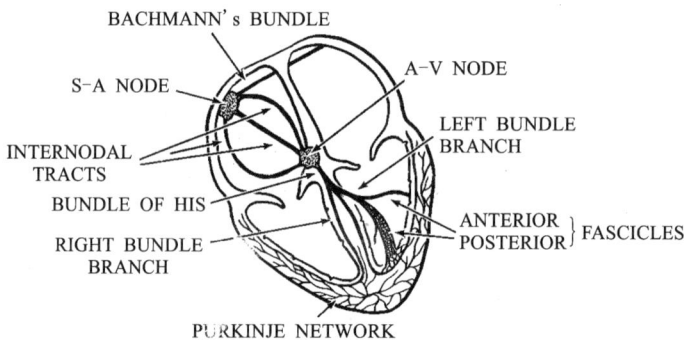

Fig. 5 – 21

(下面的章节"心室内差异性传导"是由 Alan Lindsay, Frank Yanowitz 和 J. Douglas Ridges 博士在 1980 年描述的, 在此仅作了少部分修改。)

5.3 心室内差异性传导

5.3.1 简介

室内差异性传导（AVC）是解析 12 导联心电图及其节律时经常遇到的容易让人混淆的根源。因此, 彻底弄懂和理解其发生机制并且能识别它, 是所有阅读心电图的人应该具备的基本技能。

在我们理解室内差异性传导之前, 我们必须先复习一下电冲动在心脏内的再次传导(图 5 - 21)。多么完美的设计! 来自快速自律中心(窦房结)的电脉冲兴奋并通过心房, 通过特殊的纤维(巴赫曼束传导到左心房和 3 个结间束)传导到房室结。房室结提供了足够的时间延迟来保证心房收缩和心室充盈。在缓慢的房室传导之后是高速的传导路将电脉冲传至右心室和左心室(经过希氏束, 束支及其分支, 然后到浦氏纤维网)。两个心室同时兴奋产生一个**窄的、正常的 QRS 波**(QRS 间期 0.06 ~ 0.1 s)。那么, 如果有一个束支发生传导延缓或阻滞, 就可以产生一个**异常的、宽大的 QRS 波群**[左束支的分支如果发生传导延缓或阻滞也可以产生一个异常的 QRS 波群, 虽然不是很宽大, 但是和正常的 QRS 形态不同(如额面的 QRS 电轴改变)]。

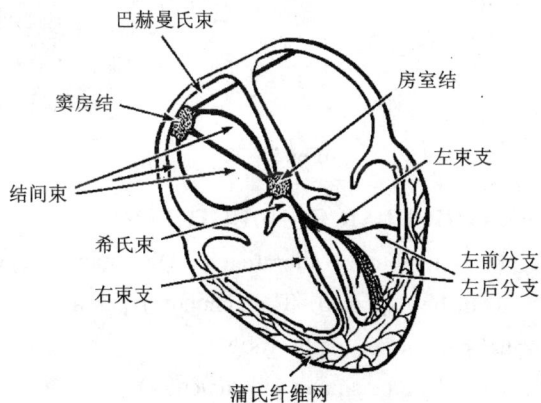

图 5 - 21

5.3.2 Fig. 5 – 22 below illustrates a basic principle of AVC. AVC is atemporary alteration of QRS morphology when you would have expected a normal QRS complex. Permanent bundle branch block (BBB) is NOT AVC.

In this discussion we will concentrate on AVC through normal bundle branch and fascicular pathways and not consider conduction through accessory pathways (e. g. , as in WPW syndrome). The ECG illustrated in Fig. 5 – 22 from lead V1 shows two normal sinus beats followed by a premature atrial complex (PAC, first arrow). The QRS complex of the PAC is narrow resembling the normal QRS morphology. After an incomplete pause, another sinus beat is followed by a slightly earlier PAC. Now, because of this slightly increased prematurity (and the longer preceding RR cycle), the QRS morphology is abnormal (rsR′ morphology of RBBB). If you were not careful you might mistake this wide funny looking beat (FLB) as a PVC and attach a different clinical significance (and therapy). The diagram on p42 also illustrates the different "fates" of PACs. The key features to recognizing AVC in this tracing are：

(1)Finding the premature P-wave (P′) or Cherchez le P (in French)

(2)Recognizing the typical RBBB QRS morphology (rsR′ in lead V1)

Lead V1

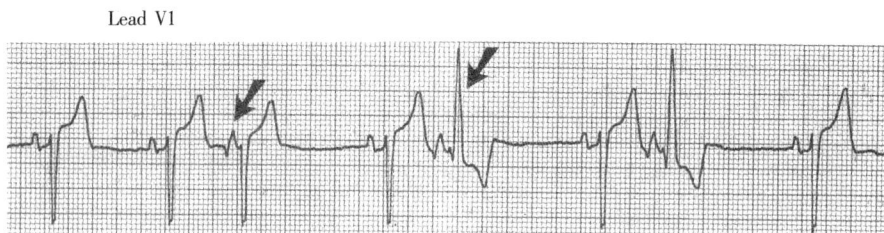

Fig. 5 – 22

ABERRANT VENTRICULAR CONDUCTION

A term that describes temporary alteration of QRS morphology under conditions where a normal QRS might be expected. The common types are：

(1)Through normal conduction pathways：

• Cycle-length dependent (Ashman phenomenon)

• Rate-dependent tachycardia or bradycardia

5.3.2 图 5-22 描述了 AVC 的基本原则。AVC 是临时改变了预期正常 QRS 波群的变形的 QRS 波群。永久束支阻滞（BBB）**不是 AVC。**

此讨论，我们将专注于 AVC 通过正常束支及其分支的传导，不认为通过辅助途径旁路传导（如 WPW 综合征）。如图 5-22 所示的心电图，V1 导联显示了两个正常窦性之后紧随 1 个心房性期前收缩（PAC，第一个箭头）。PAC 后面是窄 QRS 波群类似正常 QRS 形态，不完全间歇之后。另一个窦性后面是一个较早的 PAC。现在，由于这种稍微提前（以及之前有长 RR 周期），QRS 形态出现了异常（rsR′ RBBB 的形态）。如果你不小心，你可能错误的认为这宽大畸形的 QRS 是室性期前收缩（PVC），从而会导致不同的临床意义（和治疗）。P43 的图也说明了房性期前收缩的不同"命运"。这种识别 AVC 的关键特征是来跟踪：

（1）发现过早的 P 波（P′）或"寻找 P"（法语）。

（2）能够认识典型 RBBB 的 QRS 形态（V1 导联的 rsR′）。

V1 导联

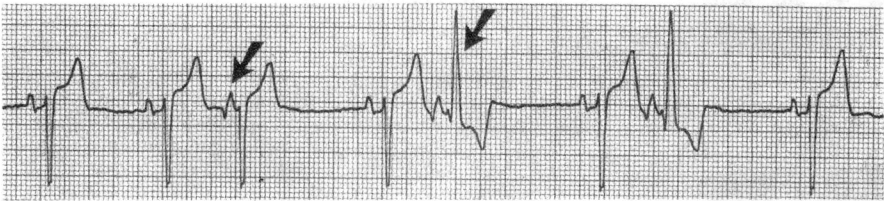

图 5-22

室内差异性传导这一术语指在应该出现正常 QRS 的地方出现了暂时的改变了形态的 QRS 波群，常见的类型是：

（1）通过正常传导通路

- 长周期依赖（Ashman 现象）。
- 心动过速或过缓的频率依赖。

(2)Through accessory pathways (e. g., Kent bundle)

As seen below five features or clues help identify AVC of theright bundle branch block variety. It should be emphasized that although RBBB morphology is the commonest form of AVC, LBBB or block of one of its fascicles may also occur, particularly in persons with more advanced left heart disease or those taking cardiovascular drugs. In healthy people the right bundle branch has a slightly longer refractory period than the left bundle at normal heart rates and, therefore, is more likely to be unavailable when an early PAC enters the ventricles. The "second-in-a row" phenomenon will be illustrated later in this section.

FEATURES FAVORING RBBB ABERRANT CONDUCTION

(1)Preceding atrial activity (premature P wave)

(2)rSR′ or rsR′ morphology in lead V1

(3)qRs morphology in lead V6

(4)Same initial r wave as normal QRS complex (in lead V1)

(5)"Second-in-a-row" phenomenon

The Ashman Phenomenon is named after the late Dr. Richard Ashman who first described, in 1947, AVC of the RBBB variety in patients with atrial fibrillation. Ashman reasoned, from observing ECG rhythms in patients with a-fib, that the refractory period (during which conducting tissue is recovering and cannot be stimulated) was directly proportional to the cycle length or heart rate. The longer the cycle length (or slower the heart rate) the longer the refractory period is. In Fig. 5 – 23 a premature stimulus (PS) can be normally conducted if the preceding cycle length is of short or medium duration but will be blocked if the preceding cycle length is long. Ashman observed this in atrial fibrillation when long RR cycles were followed by short RR cycles and the QRS terminating the short RR cycle was wide in duration (looking like RBBB).

Look at the ECG rhythm strips in Fig. 3. Simultaneous Lead Ⅱ and Lead V1 are recorded. The first PAC (first arrow in V1) conducts to the ventricles with a normal QRS because the preceding cycle was of normal or medium length. The second PAC (next arrow) conducts with RBBB (rsR′ in V1) because the preceding cycle was LONGER. Both PACs have identical coupling intervals from the preceding sinus P wave. Thus, a long cycle-short cycle sequence often leads to AVC. Unfortunately this sequence helps us UNDERSTAND AVC but is not DIAGNOSTIC OF AVC. PVCs may also occur in a long cycle-short cycle sequence. It is important, therefore, to have other clues to the differential diagnosis of funny looking QRS beats (FLBs).

（2）通过旁路（如 Kent 束）

如下五个特性或线索可帮助识别右束支阻滞型的 AVC。应该强调，尽管 RBBB 形态是 AVC 中最常见的形式，但是左束支阻滞（LBBB）或其分支阻滞型也可能发生，尤其是有严重左侧心脏病的人或服用了心血管药物的人。健康的人右束支不应期比左束支稍长一些（正常的心率时），因此，提前的 PAC 进入心室时很可能右束支不能传导。"second-in-a row"现象将会在本节稍后部分作出说明。

支持 RBBB 型差异性传导的特征有：①提前的心房活动（过早 P 波）；②V1导联 rSR′ 或 rsR′ 型；③V6 导联 qRs 型；④V1 导联的初始的 r 波与正常 QRS 波群 r波一样；⑤"Second-in-a-row"现象。

阿斯曼（Ashman）现象命名于已故的理查德·阿斯曼博士，他在 1947 年首次描述了心房纤颤时出现的 RBBB 型的 AVC。他推断，从观察心房纤颤患者的心电图节律得出，不应期（在此期间传导组织正在复极，刺激无效）直接与周期长度或心率成正比。周期长度越长（或慢心率）不应期越长。在图 5－23 中一个过早的刺激（PS）可以正常传导，因为前一周期长度是短的或适中的，但是如果前面的周期长度长就会发生阻滞。他观察到，在心房纤颤中如果紧随长 RR 周期后的是短的 RR 周期，那么短周期 RR 的 QRS 是宽大畸形的（看起来像 RBBB）。

如图 5－23 的心电图所示，同时记录 Ⅱ 和 V1 导联。第一个 PAC（V1 的第一个箭头）传导到心室是一个正常 QRS，因为前面的周期是正常的或中等长度的。第二个 PAC（第二个箭头）传导呈 RBBB 型（V1 导联是 rsR′），因为前面的周期更长。同样是房性期前收缩而且与前面窦性 P 波有相同的联律间期，只是前面的RR 周期长短不同，导致了室内差异性传导 AVC。不幸的是这个序列可以帮助我们了解 AVC 但不是诊断 AVC。因为室性期前收缩（PVC）也可能出现在一个长短周期序列。因此，重要的是要有其他线索才能对宽大畸形的 QRS（FLBs）作出鉴别诊断。

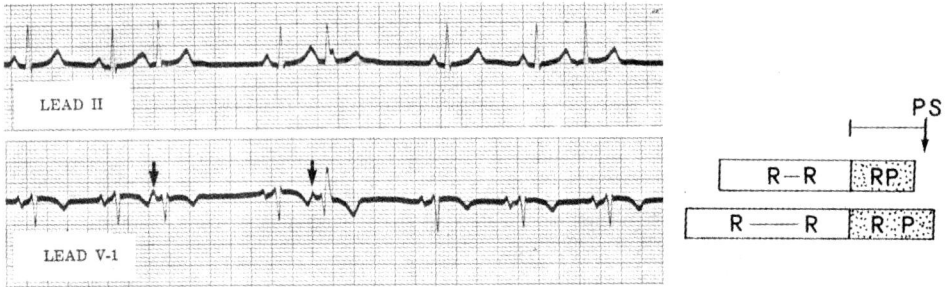

Fig. 5 – 23

Years ago Dr. Henry Marriott, a master teacher of electrocardiography and author of many outstanding ECG textbooks offered valuable guidelines regarding aberrant QRS morphologies (especially in lead V1). These morphologies contrasted with the QRS complexes often seen with PVCs and enhanced our ability to diagnose AVC. For example, if the QRS in lead V1 is predominately up-going or positive (Fig. 5 – 24) the differential diagnosis is between RBBB aberrancy and ventricular ectopy usually originating in the left ventricle. A careful look at each of the 5 QRS morphologies in Fig. 5 – 24 will identify the "Las Vegas" betting odds of making the right diagnosis.

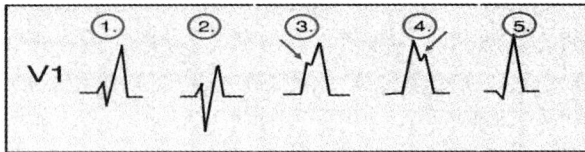

Fig. 4

QRS #1 and #2 in Fig. 5 – 24 are "classic" RBBB morphologies with rsR′ or rSR′ triphasic QRS shapes. When either of these is seen in a V1 premature beat we can be at least 90% certain that they are aberrant RBBB conduction and not ventricular ectopy. Examples #3 and #4 are notched or slurred monophasic R wave QRS complexes. Where's the notch or slur? Think of rabbit ears. If the notch or slur is on the downstroke of the QRS (little right rabbit ear in Example #4), then the odds are almost 100-to-1 that the beat is a ventricular ectopic beat (or PVC). If, on the other hand, the notch or slur is on the upstroke of the QRS (little rabbit ear on the left in Example #3), than the odds are 50 : 50 and not helpful in the differential Dx. Finally if the QRS complex has just a qR configuration (Example #5) than the odds are reasonably high that the beat in question is a ventricular ectopic beat and not AVC. Two exceptions to this last rule (#5) need to be remembered. Some people with normal ECG's do not have an initial little r-wave in the QRS of lead V1. If RBBB occurs in such a person the QRS morphology in V1 will be a qR instead of an rsR′. Secondly, in a person with a previous anterior or anteroseptal infarction the V1 QRS often has a QS morphology, and RBBB in such a person will also have a qR pattern.

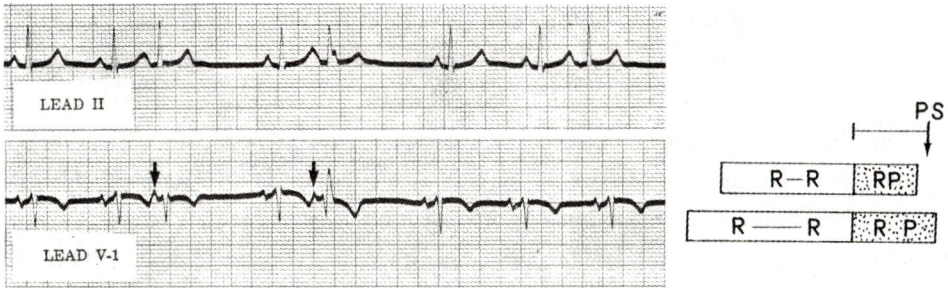

不应期（RP）随 R－R 延长而延长

图 5－23

数年前亨利·万豪博士，心电图大师，也是许多著名心电图教科书的作者，对于阅读宽大畸形的 QRS 波提供了有价值的指导方针（尤其是 V1 导联）。将这些形态的 QRS 与我们通常见到的 PVCs 波群对比，增强了我们诊断 AVC 的能力。例如，如果 V1 导联的 QRS 是明显的或正向波（图 5－24），就需要在 RBBB 型差异性传导与起源于左心室的异位搏动相鉴别。仔细看图 5－24 中每个 QRS 形态，就会知道"拉斯维加斯"赌博赔率是多少了。

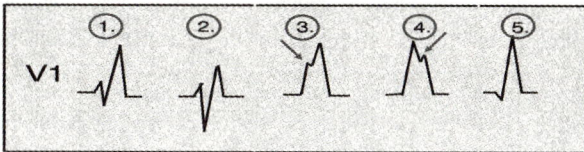

图 5－24

图 5－24 示例#1 和#2 是"经典"RBBB 形态伴有三相的 QRS 形状。当我们在 V1 导联见到这样的期前收缩时，至少 90% 可以确信他们是异常的 RBBB 差异性传导，而不是室性异位搏动。示例#3 和#4 是有切迹或顿挫 QRS 波群。切口或顿挫在哪里？想象一下兔子的耳朵，如果切迹或顿挫在 QRS 的下降支（示例#4 小兔子右耳朵），就有很大的可能几乎 100∶1 的比例是心室期前收缩（PVC）。另一方面，如果切迹或顿挫在 QRS 的上升支（左边的小兔子的耳朵在示例#3），则胜算达到 50%，而不是有助于鉴别。最后，如果 QRS 波群起始部是 qR 型（例#5），那么是一个心室异位搏动（PVC），而不是室内差异性传导（AVC）的可能性相当高。但是#5 有两个例外需要记住，有些正常人心电图 V1 导联 QRS 没有一个初始小 r 波。如果 RBBB 发生在这样的一个人身上，在 V1 导联的 QRS 形态将是 qR，而不是 rsR′。其次，如果一个人过去有过前间隔或后间隔梗死，V1 的 QRS 经常是 QS 形，如果伴有 RBBB 就会是 qR 型。

Now consider mostly down-going or negative QRS morphologies in lead V1（Fig. 5
－25）. Here the differential diagnosis is between LBBB aberration（Example #1）and
right ventricular ectopy（Example #2）. Typical LBBB in lead V1 may or may not have
a "thin" initial r-wave, but will always have a rapid S-wave downstroke as seen in #1.
On the other hand any one of three features illustrated in #2 is great betting odds that
the beat in question is ventricular ectopy and not AVC. These three features are：1）fat
little initial r-wave, 2）notch or slur in the downstroke of the S wave, 3）a 0.06 sec or
more delay from the beginning of the QRS to the nadir of the S wave.

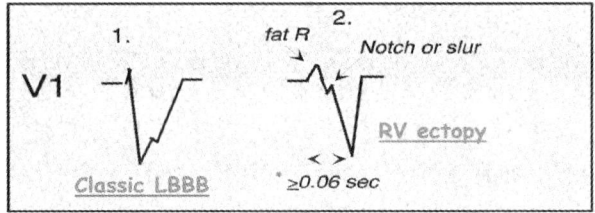

Fig. 5－25

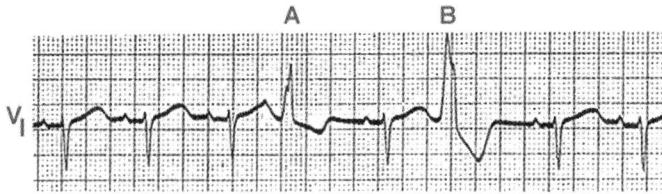

Can you differentiate sore thumbs "A" and "B"

Fig. 5－26

Now, let's look at some real ECG examples of the preceding QRS morphology
rules. We will focus on the V1 lead for now since it is the best lead for differentiating
RBBB from LBBB, and right ventricular ectopy from left ventricular ectopy.

Fig. 5 － 26 illustrates two premature funny-looking beats（FLBs）for your
consideration. FLB "A" has a small notch on the upstroke of the QRS complex
resembling #3 in Fig. 5 － 24. Remember, that's only a 50：50 odds for AVC and
therefore not helpful in the differentiating it from a PVC. However, if you look carefully
at the preceding T wave, you will see that it is more pointed than the other T wave in
this V1 rhythm strip. There is very likely a hidden premature P-wave in the T before
"A", making the FLB a PAC with RBBB aberrancy. Dr. Marriott likes to say：
"Cherchez le P" which is a sexy way to say in French "Search for the P" before the
FLB to determine if the FLB is a PAC with AVC. FLB "B", on the other hand, has a
small notch or slur on the downstroke of the QRS resembling #4 in Fig. 5 － 24. That's
almost certainly a PVC.

现在再研判一下 V1 导联 QRS 的负向波形态变化(图 5 – 25)。这主要用于鉴别 LBBB 型差异性传导(例#1)和右心室异位搏动(例#2)。典型 LBBB 在 V1 导联可能会有或可能不会有一个"瘦"初始 r 波,但是总是会有一个快速向下的 S 波(见#1)。另一方面,如果有#2 所示波形中的三个特征中任何一个,提示很可能是室性异位搏动(PVC)而不是 LBBB 型差异性传导(AVC)。这三个特点是:①肥胖的初始 r 波;②向下的 S 波有切迹或顿挫;③QRS 起始部到 S 波最低点≥0.06 s。

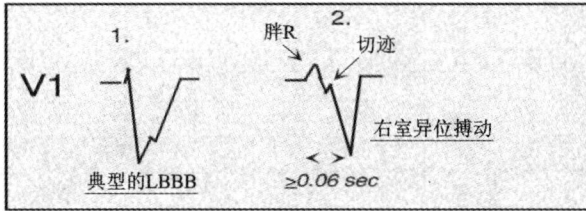

典型的 LBBB 和右心室异位搏动的鉴别

图 5 – 25

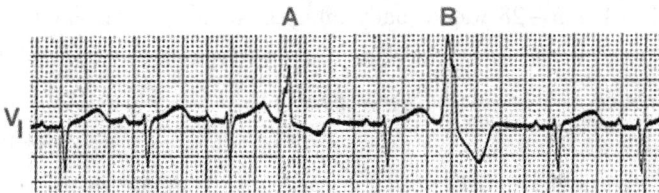

图 5 – 26

现在,让我们来看看一些真正的,之前描述过的关于 QRS 形态规则的心电图的例子。我们现在将集中在 V1 导联,因为它是区分 RBBB 和 LBBB,以及区分来自右心室和左心室异位搏动最好的导联。

图 5 – 26 演示了两个畸形(FLBs)的期前收缩供你考虑。FLB "A" 在 QRS 波群的上升支有一个小切迹,和图 5 – 24 中的#3 类似。记住,这只是一个 50∶50 AVC 的概率,因此无助于和 PVC 区分。然而,如果你仔细看前面的 T 波,你会发现它前面的 T 波比 V1 导联中的其他 T 波更尖锐一些。很有可能在这个畸形(FLBs)前面隐藏了一个过早 P 波,所以 FLB 就是 PAC 伴 RBBB 型差异性传导。万豪博士喜欢说"**Cherchez le P**",这是法语用一个性感的方式说去"**寻找 P**",如果找到了,这个畸形 FLB 就是房性期前收缩 PAC 伴差异性传导 AVC。再看另一个 FLB"B"在 QRS 的下降支有一个小切迹(如图 5 – 24 的#4 所示),当然这几乎就是一个室性期前收缩(PVC)。

Alas, into each life some rain must fall! Remember life is not always 100% perfect. In Fig. 5 – 27, after 2 sinus beats, a bigeminal rhythm develops. The 3 premature FLBs have TYPICAL RBBB MORPHOLOGY (rSR′) and yet they are PVCs! How can we tell? They are not preceded by premature P-waves, but are actually followed (look in the ST segment) by the next normal sinus P-wave which cannot conduct because the ventricles are refractory at that time. The next P wave comes on time (complete pause). Well, you can't win them all!

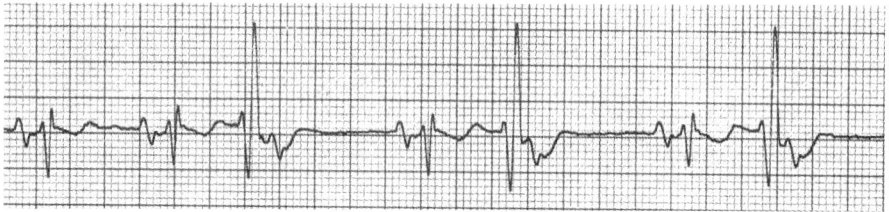

Fig. 5 – 27

The ECG in Fig. 5 – 28 was actually interpreted as "Ventricular bigeminy" in our ECG lab by a tired physician reading late at night. Try to see if you can do better. The first thing to notice is that all the early premature FLBs have RBBB morphology... already a 10 : 1 odds favoring AVC. Note also that some the T waves of the sinus beats look "funny" – particularly in Leads 1, 2, and V2. They are small, short, and peak too early, a very suspicious signal that they are, indeed, hidden premature P-waves in the T waves (Cherchez-le-P).

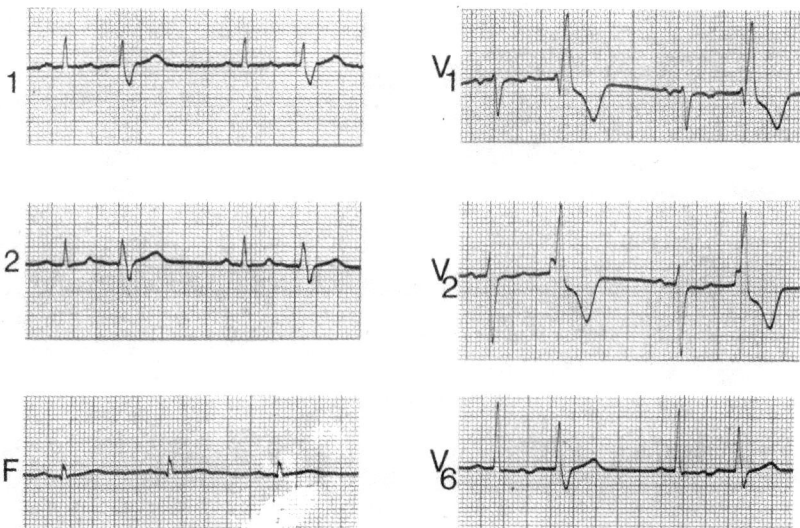

Fig. 5 – 28

唉，每个人一生都得逢上阴雨！记住生活并不总是 100% 完美的。在图 5-27 中，2 个窦性搏动过后，成对的节奏（二联律）发生了。3 个畸形 FLBs 的期前收缩是**典型 RBBB 型**（rSR′），但他们是室性期前收缩（PVC）！怎么说呢？他们不是因为之前有房性期前收缩而发生，而且实际上跟在后面的正常窦性 P 波不能下传（看看它的 ST 段），因为心室还处在不应期。下一个 P 波准时到达（完全性代偿间歇）。好，你不能总赢！

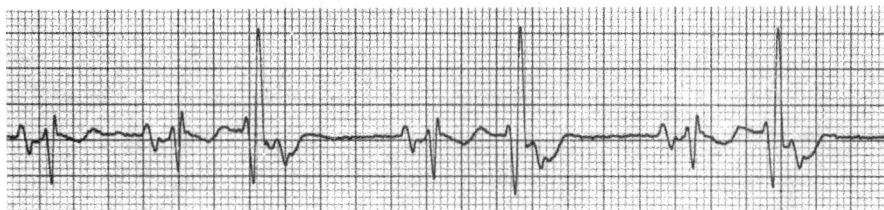

图 5-27

图 5-28 中的心电图，一位疲劳的夜班医师在心电图室解释为"室性早搏二联律"，试着看看你是否可以做得更好。首先要注意的是，所有的畸形期前收缩 FLBs 都是 RBBB 形态……已经支持了有 10:1 的可能是 AVC。还要注意一些窦性 T 波看起来很"有趣"——尤其是在 Ⅰ、Ⅱ 导联和 V2 导联。T 波有一个小，短而且提前的峰，一个非常可疑的信号，实际上，是藏在 T 波里的过早 P 波（寻找-P）。

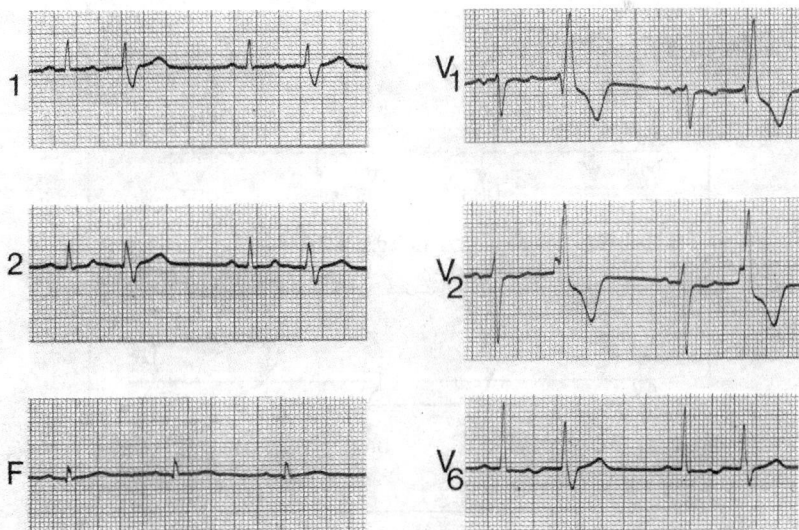

图 5-28

The clincher, however, is that the premature beats are followed by INCOMPLETE COMPENSATORY PAUSES. How can you tell? One lead (aVF) has no premature FLBs, so you can measure the exact sinus rate. Taking 2 sinus cycles from this lead (with your calipers), you can now tell in the other leads that the P wave following the FLBs comes earlier than expected suggesting that the sinus cycle was reset by the premature P waves (a common feature of PACs, but not PVCs). The correct diagnosis, therefore, is atrial bigeminy with RBBB aberration of the PACs.

As discussed on p62, the diagram illustrated in Fig. 5 – 29 helps us understand the difference between a "complete" compensatory pause (characteristic of most PVCs) and an "incomplete" pause (typical of most PACs). The top half of Fig. 5 – 29 shows (in "ladder" diagram form) three sinus beats and a PAC. The sinus P wave after the PAC comes earlier than expected because the PAC entered the sinus node and reset its timing. In the bottom half of Fig. 9 three sinus beats are followed by a PVC. As you can see the sinus cycle is not interrupted, but one sinus beat cannot conduct to the ventricles because the ventricles are refractory due to the PVC. The next P wave comes on time making the pause a complete compensatory pause.

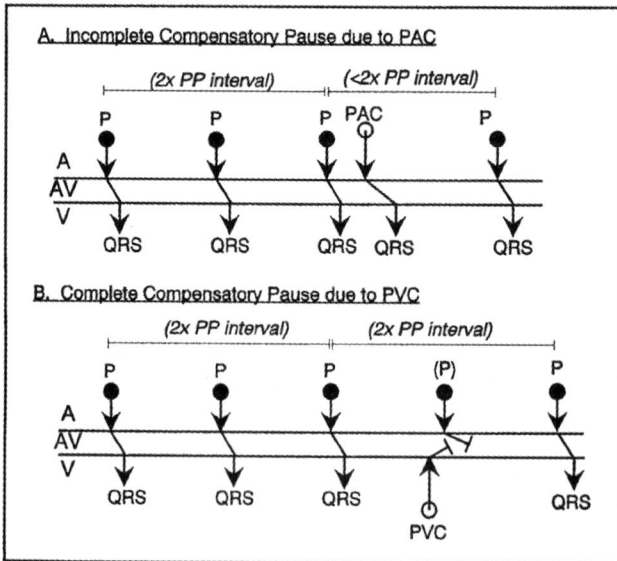

Fig. 5 – 29

然而，最关键的是，期前收缩后面的是**不完全的代偿间歇**。你怎么看出来的？一个导联（aVF）没有过早 FLBs，所以你可以准确地测量窦率，从这个导联的 2 个窦性周期（用你的卡尺）与其他有期前收缩的导联的 2 个周期比较，现在你可以知道其他导联 FLBs 前面的 P 波比预期来得早，而且窦性周期被这个期前收缩重置了（房性期前收缩 PAC 的一个常见特性，但不是室性期前收缩 PVC）。因此，正确的诊断是房性期前收缩二联律伴 RBBB 型的差异性传导。

正如在本书第 63 页所讨论的，图 5 - 29 会帮助我们理解"完全"代偿间歇（PVC 的特点）和一个"不完全"代偿间歇（典型的大多数 PAC）的区别。图 5 - 29 显示的上半部分（"阶梯"图）为 3 个窦性周期和 1 个房性期前收缩 PAC。PAC 后窦 P 波比预期来得早，因为 PAC 进入窦房结并将其时钟重置。在图 5 - 29 的下半部分为 3 个窦性周期后面有 1 个室性期前收缩 PVC。正如你所看到的，窦性周期不会被打断，但 1 个窦性周期是无法传到心室的，这是由于 PVC 所致的心室不应期。下一个 P 波准时到达可形成一个完全的代偿间歇。

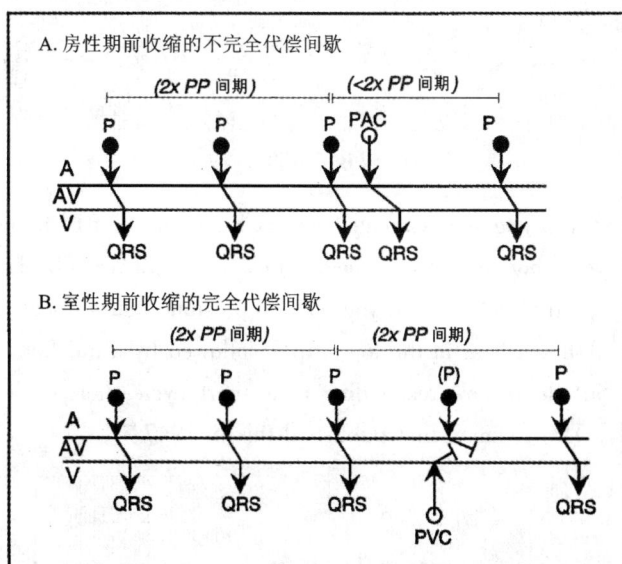

图 5 - 29

The top ECG strip in Fig. 5 – 30 illustrates 2 PACs conducted with AVC. Note how the premature ectopic P-wave peaks and distorts the preceding T-wave (Cherchez-le-P). The first PAC conducts with LBBB aberrancy and the second with RBBB. In the second strip atrial fibrillation is initiated by a PAC with RBBB aberration (note the long preceding RR interval followed by a short coupling interval to the PAC). The aberrantly conducted beat that initiates atrial fibrillation is an example of the "second-in-a-row" phenomenon which is frequently seen in atrial tachyarrhythmias with AVC. It's the second beat in a sequence of fast beats that is most often conducted with AVC because of the long-short rule (Ashman phenomenon).

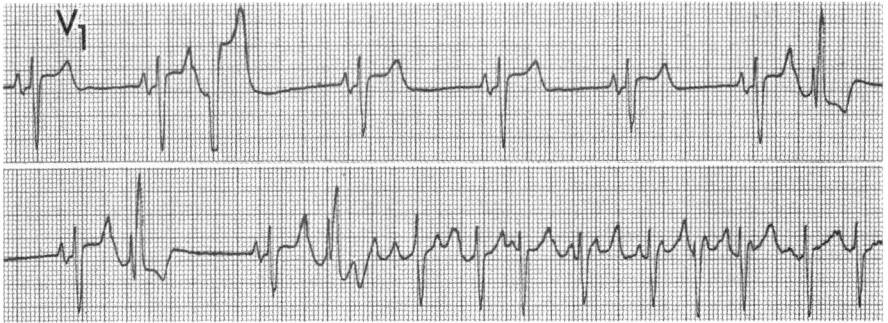

Fig. 5 – 30

In Fig. 5 – 31 you can see Ashman beats at their finest. RBBB beats in lead V1 follow the long cycle-short cycle sequence. Since the atria are fibrillating, you can't identify "preceding atrial activity" so you have to presume that all beats are conducted. Note that the 2nd Ashman beat in the top strip is followed by a quicker but narrow QRS beat – the right bundle is now responding to a short cycle-short cycle sequence and behaves normally. Dr. Ashman first published this in 1947!

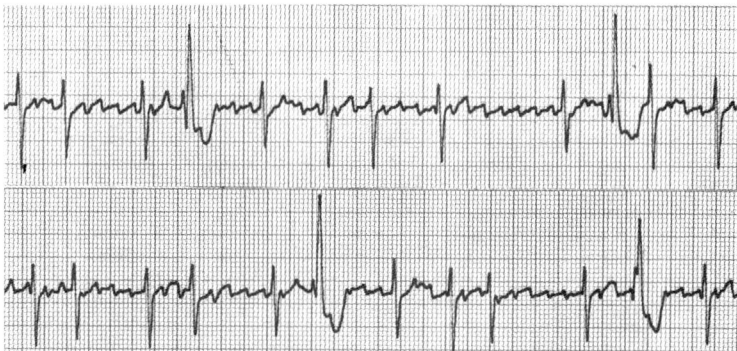

Fig. 5 – 31

图 5-30 顶端的心电图是 2 个房性期前收缩伴差异性传导。请注意之前过早的异位 P 波之峰扭曲了前面的 T 波（寻找 P）。第一个 PAC 伴 LBBB 型差异性传导，第二个伴 RBBB 型差异性传导。第二条心电图是由一个伴 RBBB 型差异性传导的房性期前收缩 PAC 引起的心房纤颤（注意前面的 RR 间期是长的，后面跟着一个短的房性期前收缩 PAC 的联律间期）。这个伴有差异性传导的期前收缩诱发了心房纤颤，"second-in-a-row"现象是房性快速心律失常的一个常见的例子。这个快频率的第二跳通常引起差异性传导，遵循了长短周期原则（阿斯曼现象）。

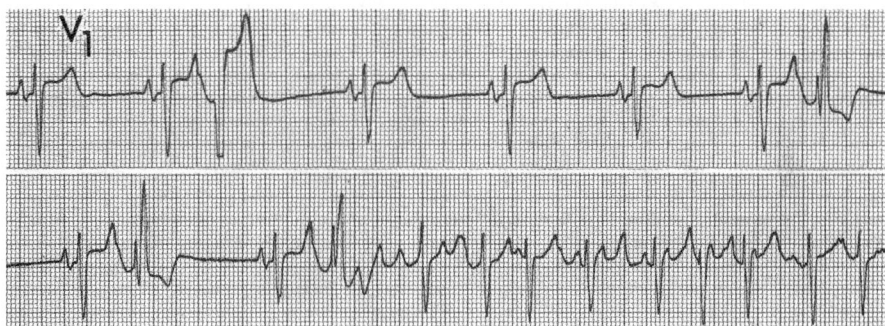

图 5-30

在图 5-31 中可以看到最好的阿斯曼现象。V1 导联中 RBBB 波出现在长周期后。由于心房纤颤，你不能确定"前面的心房活动"，所以你必须假定所有的心房纤颤波都能传导。注意第二个阿斯曼搏动后面跟随 1 个更快但窄的 QRS 波群，说明此时的右束支对应的是短周期顺序，所以其行为（不应期）正常。阿斯曼博士在 1947 年首次出版发布了这一点！

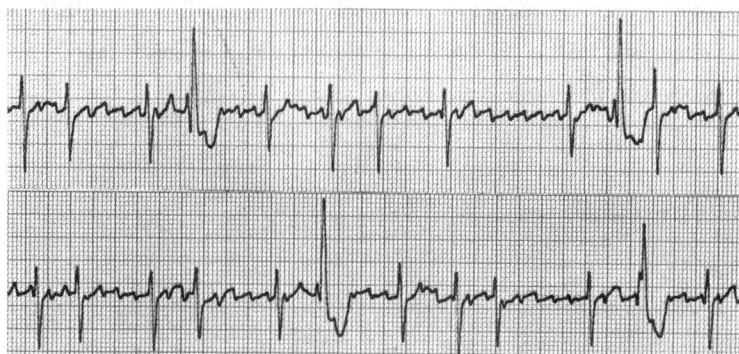

图 5-31

If you're ready for some fun, consider the next example illustrated in Fig. 5 – 32. This unfortunate man suffered from palpitations and dizziness when he swallowed. What you see is an ectopic atrial tachycardia with intermittent RBBB aberrant conduction. The arrows point to ectopic P-waves firing at nearly 200 bpm. Note how the PR interval gradually gets longer until the 4th ectopic P-wave in the tachycardia fails to conduct (Wenckebach phenomenon). This initiates a pause (longer cycle), and when 1：1 conduction resumes the second and subsequent QRS complexes exhibit upright QRS complexes in the form of atypical RBBB. This has to be a truly cool ECG rhythm strip! The man was told to stop swallowing!

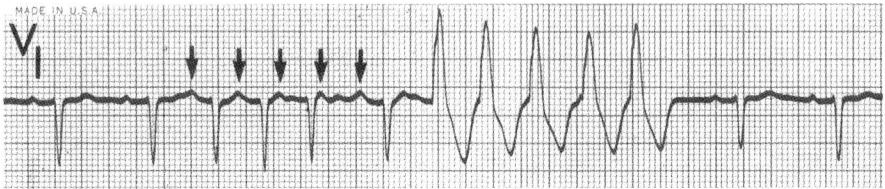

Fig. 5 – 32

Bundle branch block aberration can occur during a "critical rate" change which means that AVC comes with gradual changes in heart rate and not necessarily with abrupt changes in cycle length as in the Ashman phenomenon. Think of a "tired" but not "dead" bundle branch. This is illustrated in Fig. 5 – 33 (lead Ⅱ), an example of rate-dependent or acceleration-dependent AVC. When the sinus cycle, in this instance 71 bpm, is shorter than the refractory period of the left bundle then LBBB ensues. It is almost always the case that as the heart rate slows it takes a slower rate for the LBBB to disappear, as seen in the lower strip.

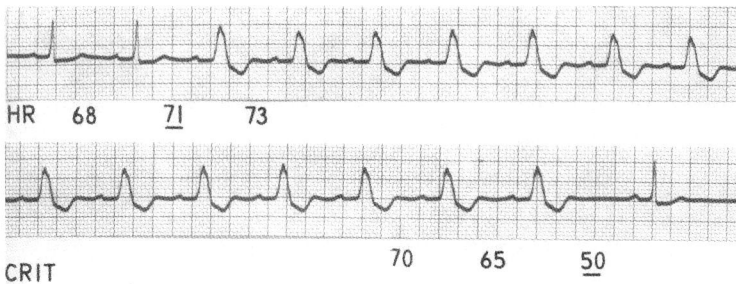

Fig. 5 – 33

如果你准备要了解一些有趣的,可以考虑下一个示例(如图5-32所示)。这个不幸的人当他吞咽时患有心悸,头晕,你看到的是一个异位房性心动过速与间歇RBBB型差异性传导。箭头所指的异位P波以接近200次/min频率起搏。注意PR间期逐渐延长,直到第4个异位P不能下传(文氏现象),这启动了一个暂停(长周期),当1:1传导恢复时,随后的第二个QRS表现出正向直立的QRS——非典型RBBB的形式,产生了差异性传导。这是一条真正的酷的心电图!这个人被告知要停止吞咽!

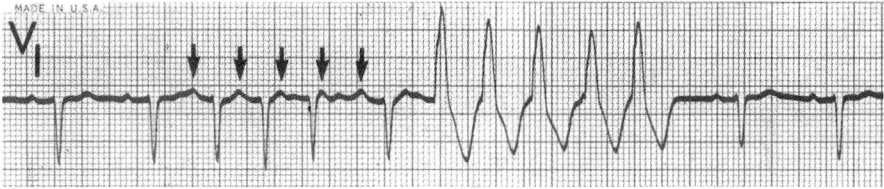

图5-32

束支阻滞型差异性传导也可发生在一个"临界频率"变化时,就是说,差异性传导产生于心率逐渐变化,而并不一定是像阿斯曼现象那样产生于周期的突然变化。束支"累了"但没有"死",如图5-33所示(Ⅱ导联)是一个频率依赖型或速度依赖型室内差异性传导的例子。当心率为71次/min时,窦性周期短于左束支的不应期,LBBB型差异性传导就发生了。它几乎总是如此,随着心率减慢,就消失了,见图5-33。

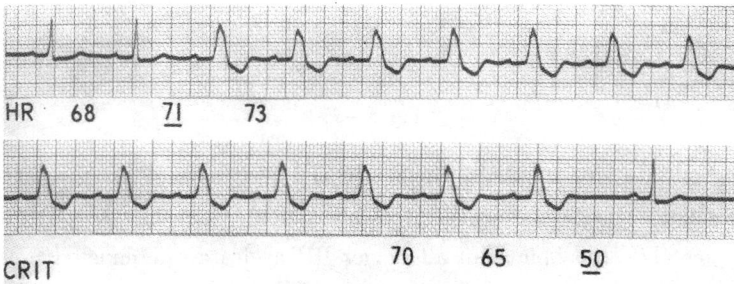

图5-33

Fig. 5 – 34 shows another example of acceleration-dependent RBBB, this time in the setting of atrial fibrillation. Even the "normal" beats have a minor degree of incomplete RBBB (rsr'). At critically short cycles, however, complete RBBB ensues and remains until the rate slows again. You can tell that these are not PVCs and runs of ventricular tachycardia because of the typical RBBB morphology (rsR' in lead V1) and the irregular RR cycles of atrial fib.

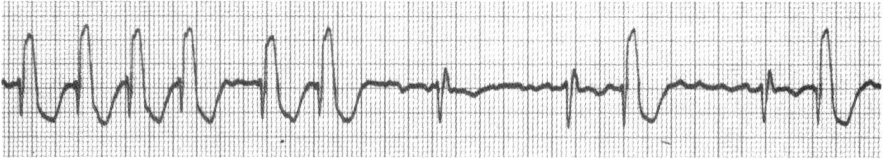

Fig. 5 – 34

Things can really get scary in the coronary care unit in the setting of acute myocardial infarction. Consider the case illustrated in Fig. 5 – 35 (lead V1) with intermittent runs of what looks like ventricular tachycardia. Note that the basic rhythm is irregularly irregular indicating atrial fibrillation. The wide QRS complexes are examples of tachycardia-dependent LBBB aberration, not runs of ventricular tachycardia. Note the morphology of the wide beats. Although there is no initial "thin" r-wave, the downstroke of the S wave is very rapid (see #1 in Fig. 5 – 35).

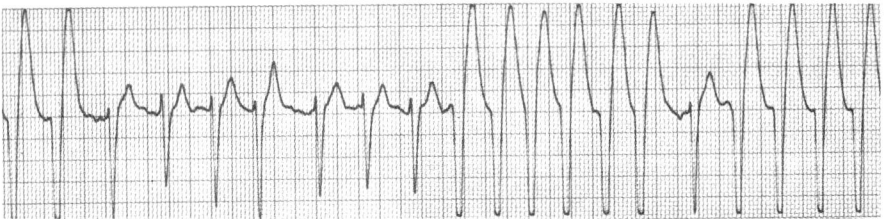

Fig. 5 – 35

Finally we have an example in Fig. 5 – 36 of a very unusual and perplexing form of AVC-deceleration or bradycardia-dependent aberration. Note that the QRS duration is normal at rates above 65 bpm, but all longer RR cycles are terminated by beats with LBBB. What a paradox! You have to be careful not to classify the late beats ventricular escapes, but in this case the QRS morphology of the late beats is classic for LBBB (see #1 in Fig. 5 – 25) as evidenced by the "thin" r-wave and rapid downstroke of the S-wave. This type of AVC is sometimes called "Phase 4" AVC because it's during Phase 4 of the action potential that latent pacemakers (in this case located in the left bundle) begin to depolarize. Sinus beats entering the partially depolarized left bundle conduct more slowly and sometimes are nonconducted (resulting in LBBB).

让我们来看看一个更迷人的心电图（图 5 - 38），这个心电图看上去很滑稽可笑。在这个 12 导心电图中有 4 个房性期前收缩（ECG 底部 V1 导联最清楚），箭头指向 4 个房性期前收缩的每一个（3 个隐藏在 T 波里）。第 1 个房性期前收缩 PAC 在 V1 导联是 qR 形，提示一个不典型 RBBB（图 5 - 24 中#5）。缺乏一个初始的"r"波是因为窦性跳动在 V1 导联就没有初始的"r"波。还要注意，在 I、II、III 导联中第一个房性期前收缩的 QRS 有明显的电轴左偏（明显向左的力量）表明是左前分支阻滞型差异性传导。V1 导联的第二个房性期前收缩隐藏在前面的 T 波里，表现为 LBBB 型的 AVC（图 5 - 25 中的#1）伴有快速下降的 QRS 波群。第三个房性期前收缩（也隐藏在 T 波里）没有 QRS 波群跟随它，因此是**未下传的房性期前收缩**。不过它重置了窦房结时间解释了节律中的间歇。（记住：**意外暂停节奏最常见的原因是一个未下传的房性期前收缩**）。第四个房性期前收缩（见 T 波后）正常传导，因为它来得足够晚以至于传导通路已经完全恢复。**这个 12 导心电图是一个出色的三个房性期前收缩命运的例子：①正常传导；②差异性传导；③未传导**。这也说明了房性期前收缩可以出现不同形式的差异性传导包括束支以及分支的传导延迟。

虽然无关，但在图 5 - 38 中发现有趣的是在 V1 ~ V3 导联 U 波振幅增加。这是在未下传房性期前收缩后的长间歇之后第一个心搏后出现的，因为 U 波通常在心率较慢时振幅增加。注意 V1 ~ V3 导联的第二个波动的 U 波有些小，与较短的周期长度有关。本书后面的章节中会有更多关于 U 波的介绍。

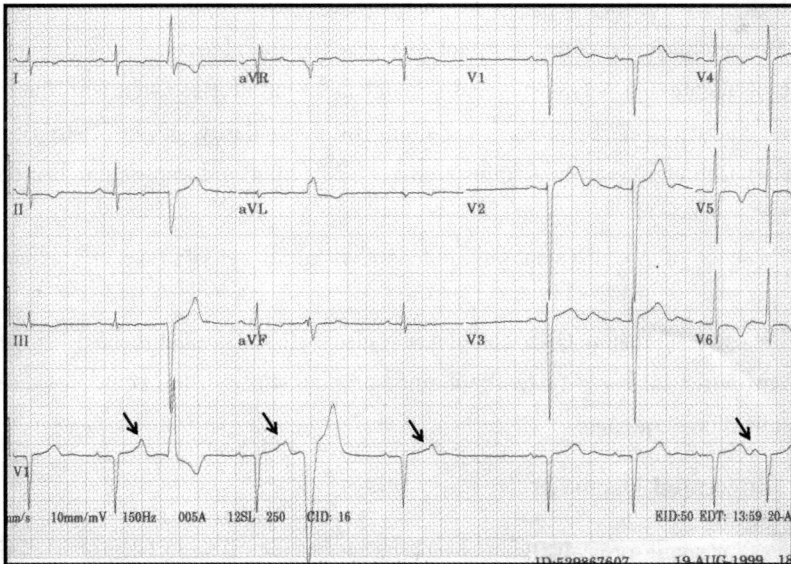

图 5 - 38

5.3.3 AVC SUMMARY

The differential diagnosis of FLBs is intellectually challenging and has important clinical implications. This section has provided clues that help distinguish wide QRS complexes that are supraventricular in origin with AVC from ectopic beats of ventricular origin (PVCs and ventricular tachycardia). When looking at single premature FLBs always search for hidden premature P-waves in the ST – T wave of the preceding beat (Cherchez-le-P). Measure with calipers the pause after the FLB to determine if it's compensatory or not. Remember the lead V1 morphology clues offered in Fig. 5 – 24 and Fig. 5 – 25 that provide the betting odds that a particular beat in question is supraventricular or ventricular in origin. These morphology clues may be the only way to correctly diagnose wide QRS-complex tachycardias.

Don't be fooled by first impressions. Not all FLBs are ventricular in origin!

5.4　Ventricular Tachycardia

This section focuses on ECG aspects of ventricular tachycardia and the differential diagnosis of wide QRS tachycardias. Other ventricular rhythms are also briefly discussed.

5.4.1　Descriptors to consider when considering ventricular tachycardia:

- Sustained (lasting > 30 s) vs. nonsustained
- Monomorphic (uniform morphology) vs. polymorphic vs. Torsades-de-pointes (Torsade-de-pointes: a polymorphic ventricular tachycardia associated with the long-QT syndromes characterized by phasic variations in the polarity of the QRS complexes around the baseline. Ventricular rate is often > 200 bpm and ventricular fibrillation is often a consequence).
- Presence of AV dissociation (independent atrial activity) vs. retrograde atrial capture
- Presence of fusion QRS complexes (also called Dressler beats) which occur when supraventricular beats (usually of sinus origin) slip into the ventricles during the ectopic activation sequence.

5.4.2　Differential Diagnosis

Just as for single premature funny-looking beats, not all wide QRS tachycardias are ventricular in origin (they may be supraventricular tachycardias with bundle branch block or WPW preexcitation)!

5.3.3 室内差异性传导小结

畸形 QRS(FLBs)的鉴别诊断是智力挑战,具有重要的临床意义。本节提供了线索,帮助区分宽 QRS 波的鉴别诊断,是室上性起源伴差异性传导还是心室异位起源搏动(PVC 或室性心动过速)的鉴别是临床难点。当看到单一畸形期前收缩时,总是要寻找隐藏在其前面的 ST – T 中的过早 P 波(寻找 P)。用游标卡尺测量畸形 QRS 后的暂停,以确定代偿间歇。对于是室上性还是室性起源难以区分的时候,记得 V1 导联形态学线索提供的图 5 – 24 和图 5 – 25 会提供诊断的几率,这些形态学线索可能是正确诊断宽 QRS 心动过速的唯一途径。

不要被第一印象蒙蔽。**不是所有畸形 QRS 波 FLBs 都起源于心室**!

5.4 室性心动过速(室性心动过速)

本节将着重于室性心动过速的心电图方面和宽 QRS 心动过速的鉴别诊断,其他心室节律也简要讨论。

5.4.1 考虑室性心动过速时要描述

- 持续性(持久 >30 s)与非持续性(<30 s)。
- 单型的(形态一致)、多型的和尖端扭转型(**尖端扭转型室性心动过速**是一种以 QT 时间延长为特征的多形态的室性心动过速,QRS 波群围绕基线不断发生相位和极性的变化,心室率往往 >200 次/min 而且通常的后果是心室颤动)。
- 存在房室分离(独立的心房活动)与逆行心房夺获。
- 存在 QRS 融合波(也叫 Dressler 搏动),当心室处在异位除极时,室上性搏动(通常窦性起源)也同时传导到心室而发生。

5.4.2 鉴别诊断

和单个的畸形的期前收缩一样,不是所有的宽 QRS 心动过速都是起源于心室(它们可能是室上性心动过速伴束支阻滞或者是 WPW 预激综合征)!

Differential Diagnosis of Wide QRS Tachycardias

(1) Although this is an ECG tutorial, let's not forget some simple bedside and clinical clues to ventricular tachycardia：

● Presence of advanced heart disease (e. g. , coronary heart disease) favors ventricular tachycardia

● Cannon "a" waves in the jugular venous pulse suggests ventricular tachycardia with AV dissociation. Under these circumstances atrial contraction from sinus rhythm may sometimes occur when the tricuspid valve is closed causing retrograde blood flow into the jugular veins (giant "a" wave).

● Variable intensity of the S1 heart sound at the apex (mitral closure) ; again this is seen when there is AV dissociation resulting in varying position of the mitral valve leaflets depending on the timing of atrial and ventricular systole.

● If the patient is hemodynamically unstable, it's probably ventricular tachycardia and act accordingly!

(2) ECG Clues：

● Regularity of the rhythm：Sustained monomorphic (all QRS's look the same) ventricular tachycardias are usually regular (i. e. , equal RR intervals) ; an irregularly-irregular wide-QRS rhythm suggests atrial fibrillation with aberration or with WPW preexcitation.

● A-V Dissociation strongly suggests ventricular tachycardia! Unfortunately AV dissociation only occurs in approximately 50% of ventricular tachycardias (the other 50% have retrograde atrial capture or "V-A association"). Of the V-techs' with AV dissociation, it can only be easily recognized if the rate of tachycardia is < 150 bpm. Faster heart rates make it difficult to find dissociated P waves.

● Fusion beats or captures often occur when there is AV dissociation and this also strongly suggests a ventricular origin for the wide QRS tachycardia.

● QRS morphology in lead V1, illustrated in Fig. 5 – 24 and Fig. 5 – 25, is often thebest clue to the origin, so go back and check out these clues! Also consider a few additional morphology clues：

· Bizarre frontal-plane QRS axis (i. e. from + 150 degrees to – 90 degrees or NW quadrant) suggests ventricular tachycardia

· QRS morphology identical to previously seen PVCs suggests ventricular tachycardia

· If all the QRS complexes from V1 to V6 are in the same direction (either all positive or all negative), ventricular tachycardia is likely

宽 QRS 心动过速的鉴别诊断如下。

(1)临床线索:虽然这是一个心电图教程,但我们不要忘记室性心动过速的一些简单的床旁的临床线索:

● 存在严重心脏病(如冠心病)倾向于室性心动过速。

● 颈静脉脉搏动可见大炮"a"波,表明室性心动过速伴房室分离。在这种情况下,来自于窦性心律的心房收缩时,可能会遇到三尖瓣关闭(心室也同时收缩)导致逆行血流入颈静脉(发生大的"a"波)。

● 心尖部 S1 心音强度发生变化(二尖瓣关闭时);这是当有房室分离时,如果心房和心室同时收缩会导致二尖瓣叶的位置变化(S1 增强)。

● 如果患者血流动力学不稳定,这可能是室性心动过速并应采取相应行动!

(2)心电图线索

● 节奏的规律性:持续单型的室性心动过速(所有的 QRS 看起来一样)通常是规则的(即相等的 RR 间隔);一个无规律又不规则的宽 QRS 节律提示心房纤颤伴差异性传导或 WPW 预激综合征。

● 房室分离强烈提示室性心动过速!不幸的是只有大约 50% 的室性心动过速发生房室分离(另外 50% 逆传夺获心房或"室房分离")。当频率 < 150 次/min 时,很容易识别出室性心动过速的房室分离,但是当频率很快时很难发现分离的 P 波。

● 融合波或心室夺获通常发生在房室分离时,这也强烈提示宽 QRS 心动过速是心室起源。

● 在 V1 导联的 QRS 形态,如图 5-24 和图 5-25 所示,通常是**最好的线索**来源,所以回去看看这些线索!还要考虑一些额外的形态学线索:

· 奇异额面 QRS 电轴(即从 +150°到 -90°或西北象限)提示室性心动过速。

· QRS 形态如果与先前出现的室性期前收缩完全相同提示室性心动过速。

· Mostly or all negative QRS morphology in V6 suggests ventricular tachycardia

· Especially wide QRS complexes（>0.16 s）suggests ventricular tachycardia

· Also consider the famousFour-Question Algorithm reported by Brugada et al, Circulation 1991；83：1649：

Step 1：Absence of RS complex in all leads V1 – V6? If Yes：Dx is ventricular tachycardia！

Step 2：No：Is interval from beginning of R wave to nadir of S wave >0.1 s in any RS lead? If Yes：Dx is ventricular tachycardia！

Step 3：No：Are AV dissociation, fusions, or captures seen? If Yes：Dx is ventricular tachycardia！

Step 4：No：Are there morphology criteria（see p72, p74）for VT present both in leads V1 and V6? If Yes：Dx is ventricular tachycardia！

If NO：Diagnosis is supraventricular tachycardia with aberration！

The ECG shown in Fig. 5 – 39 illustrates several features of typical VT：1）QRS morphology in lead V1 looks like #4 in Fig. 5 – 24, the notch is on the downstroke of the R wave；2）the QRS is mostly negative in lead V6；3）bizarre frontal plane QRS axis of − 180 degrees. This VT is most likely from the left ventricle（note the direction of QRS forces is rightward and anterior；i. e., the QRS originates in the leftward, posterior LV）.

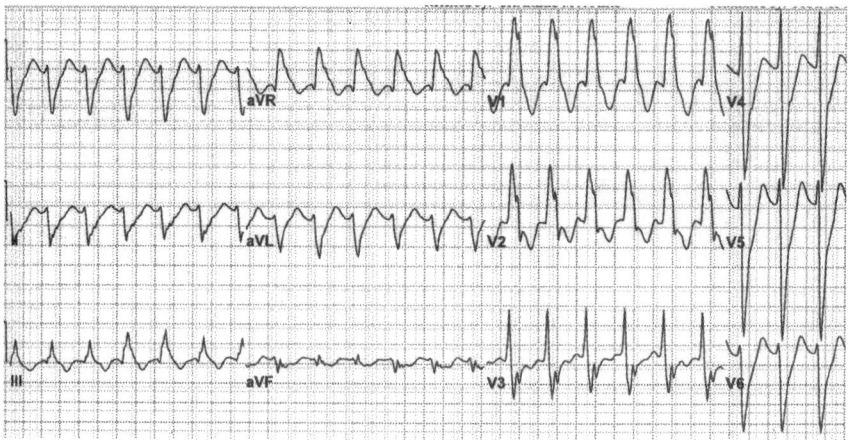

Left Ventricular Tachycardia

Fig. 5 – 39

· 如果 V1 ~ V6 导联所有的 QRS 波在同一个方向(所有都正或所有都负),室性心动过速可能性大。

· V6 导联大部分或所有的 QRS 都是负向波提示室性心动过速。

· 尤其是宽 QRS 波(>0.16 s)提示室性心动过速还要考虑 Brugada 等报道的著名的"四步问算法"(发表在循环杂志 1991；83：1649)。

步骤 1：是所有 V1 ~ V6 导联没有 RS 波吗？如果**是，提示是室性心动过速！**

步骤 2：**不是，**在任何一个有 RS 波的导联中，从 R 波起始至 S 波最低点是否 >0.1 s？如果**是，提示是室性心动过速！**

步骤 3：**不是，**存在房室分离，融合波或室性夺获吗？如果**是的，提示是室性心动过速！**

步骤 4：**不是，**V1 和 V6 导联有室性心动过速的形态学标准(见 P73，P75)吗？如果**是的，提示是室性心动过速！**

如果以上都不是，诊断为室上性心动过速伴差异性传导！

如图 5 - 39 所示的心电图显示了典型的室性心动过速(VT)的几个特点：① V1 导联 QRS 形态看起来像图 5 - 24 中的#4，R 波的降支有切迹；② V6 导联中的 QRS 大多是负的；③奇怪的是，额平面 QRS 电轴 -180°。这 VT 最有可能来自于左心室(注意 QRS 电轴的方向是向右，前；也就是说，QRS 起源于在左方，左心室后)。

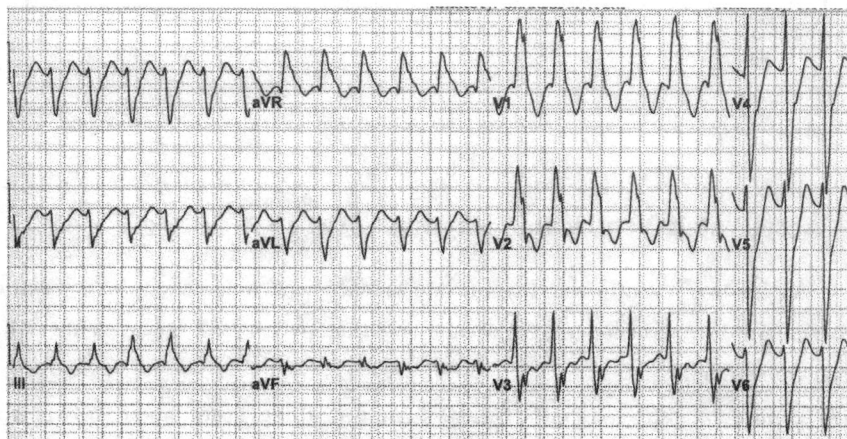

左心室心动过速

图 5 - 39

The ECG illustrated in Fig. 5 – 40 shows another typical VT, but this time originating in the right ventricle. Note the V1 QRS morphology has all the features of a right ventricular VT origin (see Fig. 5 – 25) including 1) fat, little R wave; 2) notch on the downstroke or the S-wave; and 3) >0.06 s delay from QRS onset to the nadir (bottom) of the S-wave. The direction of QRS forces is leftward and posterior (i. e., coming from a rightward and anterior RV).

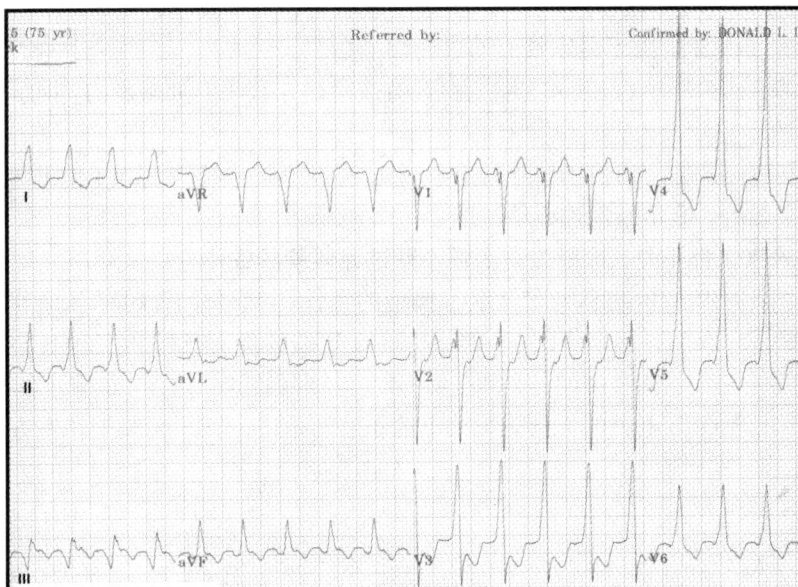

Right ventricular Tachycardia

Fig. 5 –40

5.5　Accelerated Ventricular Rhythms (see ECG in Fig. 5 –41)

- An "active" ventricular rhythm due to enhanced automaticity of a ventricular pacemaker site (reperfusion after thrombolytic therapy or PCI Rx in acute MI is a common causal factor).

- Ventricular rate can be 60 – 110 bpm (anything faster would be ventricular tachycardia).

- Sometimes this is called anisochronic ventricular rhythm when the ventricular rate is not too different from the basic sinus rate.

- May begin and end with fusion beats (ventricular activation partly due to the normal sinus activation of the ventricles and partly from the ectopic focus).

- Usually benign, short lasting and not requiring any particular therapy.

图 5 -40 所示的心电图显示另一个典型的 VT,但是这次源自右心室。注意 V1 QRS 形态有起源于右心室的 VT 的所有特性(见图 5 - 25),包括:①胖的,小 R 波;②下降支或 S 波有切迹;③从 R 波起始至 S 波最低点(底部)延迟 >0.06 s。QRS 电轴的方向向左和向后(即来自右前和右心室前壁)。

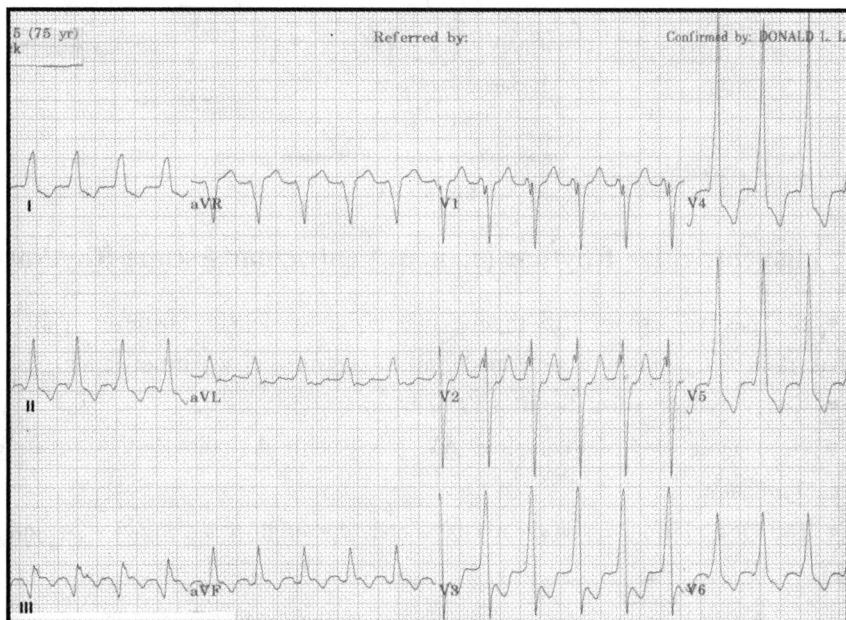

右心室心动过速

图 5 - 40

5.5 加速性室性节律

- 加速性室性节律(见图 5 - 41)是指由于心室自搏的自律性增加所表现的 "活跃"的心室节律(常见于急性心肌梗死溶栓治疗或 PCI 术后再灌注)。
- 心室率可以为 60 ~ 110 次/min(任何更快的将是室性心动过速)。
- 如果心室率和窦性频率接近,有时被称为**室性自主节律**。
- 可能以融合波开始和以融合波结束(可由正常窦房结的搏动激活部分心室,心室异位搏动激活部分心室)。
- 通常是良性的,不持久的,并不需要任何特定的治疗。

Lead MCL₁

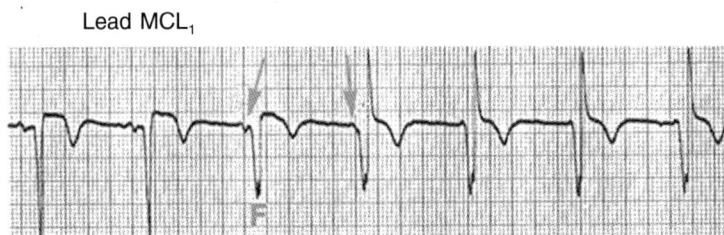

Isochronic Ventricular rhythm

F = Fusion beat

Arrows point at dissociated P waves

Fig. 5 – 41

5.6 Idioventricular Rhythm (a. k. a. Ventricular Escape Rhythm)

• A "passive" wide QRS rhythm that occursby default whenever higher-lever pacemakers in AV junction or sinus node fail to control ventricular activation.

• Escape rates are usually 30 – 50 bpm.

• Seen most often in complete AV block with AV dissociation or in other bradycardia conditions.

• The QRS morphology is clearly of ventricular origin (see Fig. 5 – 24 and Fig. 5 – 25).

5.7 Ventricular Parasystole

• Parasystolic PVCs come from protected ectopic pacemaker cells in the ventricles that fire at a fixed rate unrelated to the underlying basic rhythm (usually sinus). As a result they appear as PVCs with varying coupling intervals, and, if late enough in the cardiac cycle they may fuse with the next sinus beat).

• Non-fixed coupled PVCs where the inter-ectopic intervals (i. e. , timing between PVCs) are some multiple (i.e. , 1x, 2x, 3x, ... , etc.) of the basic rate of the parasystolic focus.

• The PVCs have uniform morphology unless fusion beats occur.

• Usuallyentrance block is present around the ectopic focus, which means that the primary rhythm (e. g. , sinus rhythm) is unable to enter the ectopic site and reset its timing.

• May also seeexit block; i. e. , the output from the ectopic site may occasionally be blocked (i. e. , no PVC when one is expected).

Lead MCL₁

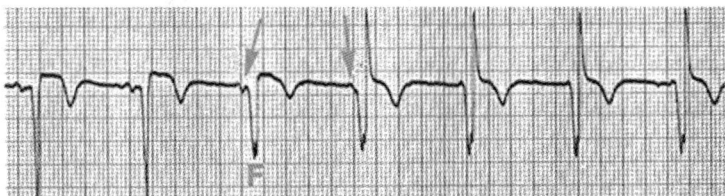

室性自主节律，F＝融合波，箭头指向房室分离的 P 波

图 5 – 41

5.6 心室自身节律

● 默认情况下只要比心室高的起搏点，包括房室结或窦房结不能控制心室兴奋时，一个"被动"的、宽 QRS 的心室节律就会产生（也称为室性逸搏律）。

● 逸搏频率一般为 30 ~ 50 次/min。

● 通常可以看到完全房室传导阻滞伴有房室分离或其他心动过缓的情况。
QRS 形态明显来源于心室（见图 5 – 24 和图 5 – 25）。

5.7 心室并行收缩（室性并行心律）

● **并行性室性期前收缩** PVCs 来自于一些受保护的心室异位起搏点细胞，它以与基本节律（通常为窦性）无关的频率起搏。结果他们表现为室性期前收缩伴有不同的耦合间隔（联律间期），如果他们在心动周期中出现的足够晚就可能与下一个窦性周期融合。

● 没有固定联律间期的室性期前收缩之间的时间间隔是并行性起搏基本频率的倍数（即 1 倍，2 倍，3 倍……）。意思是最长的室性期前收缩间隔时间可能是最短的室性期前收缩间隔时间的倍数，或两者有一个公约数。比如最长的室性期前收缩间隔是 2000 ms，最短的室性期前收缩间隔是 800ms，虽然 2000 不是 800 的整数倍数，但有一个公约数 400 ms，因此说 400 ms 很可能是室性异位起搏的自律周期，如果这个起搏点没有传出阻滞的话，就会表现为一个 150 次/min 的室性心动过速。之所以说室性并行心律来自于一些受保护的心室异位起搏点细胞是指在起搏点周围有传入阻滞，窦性节律的冲动无法进入异位起搏点和重置它的时间。但也有传出阻滞，如果没有传出阻滞，就是室性心动过速。

● PVCs 有统一的形态，除非融合波发生。

● 通常在起搏点周围有传入阻滞，这意味着主要的节律（如窦性节律）无法进入异位起搏点和重置它的时间。

● 也看到传出阻滞，即来自异位起搏点的传出冲动可能偶尔被阻滞（即在预计 PVC 出现的地方没有 PVC）。

• Fusion beats are common when the ectopic site in the ventricle fires while ventricles are already being activated from sinus pacemaker. In the rhythm in Fig. 5 – 42 non-fixed coupled PVC's are seen with fusion beats（F）. When the PVC occurs late enough in the sinus cycle they begin tofuse with the sinus beats.

• Parasystolic rhythms may also originate in the atria（i. e. , with non-fixed coupled PAC's）and within the AV junction.

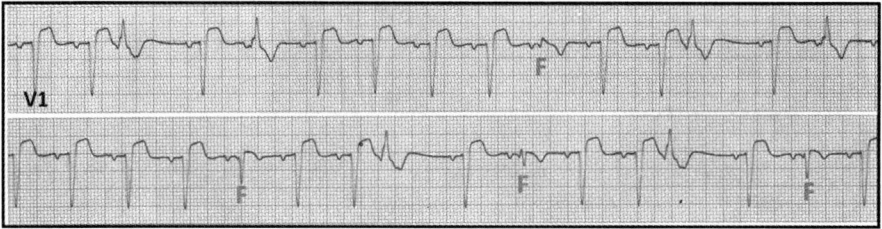

Fig. 5 – 42

5.8　Pacemaker Rhythms

Pacemakers come in a wide variety of programmable features. The following ECG rhythm strips illustrate the common types of pacing functions.

（1）Atrial pacing：note small pacemaker spikes before every P wave followed by normal QRS complexes（used mostly for sinus node disease and related bradycardias）

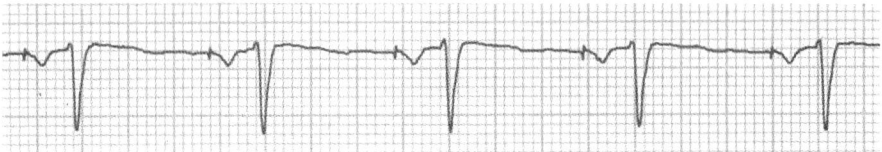

Fig. 5 – 43

（2）A-V sequential pacing with ventricular pacing（note tiny spike before each QRS）and atrialsensing of normal sinus rhythm（note：pacemaker spikes are sometimes difficult to see）：

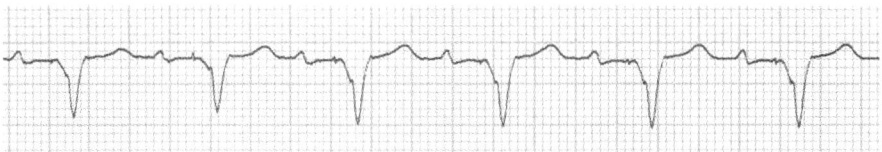

Fig. 5 – 44

（3）A-V sequential pacing with both atrial and ventricular pacing（note pacing spikes before each P wave and each QRS）：

● 融合波是常见的，因为当异位起搏点在心室起搏时，正逢窦性下传兴奋心室。在图5-42的心电图中可见到没有固定联律间期的室性期前收缩，有的伴有融合波（F）。当PVC足够晚发生在窦周期时，他们开始与窦性周期融合。

● 并行性心律也可以起源于心房[如可见联律间期不固定的房性期前收缩（PACs）]或起源于房室结。

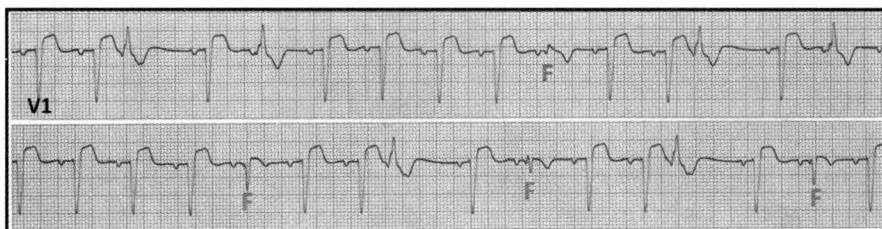

图5-42

5.8　起搏器心律

起搏器具有各种各样的可编程特性。下列心电图描述了起搏功能的常见类型。

（1）心房起搏：注意在每一个P波前有一个小的起搏标记，其后跟随正常QRS波群（主要用于窦房结疾病和相关的心动过缓）。

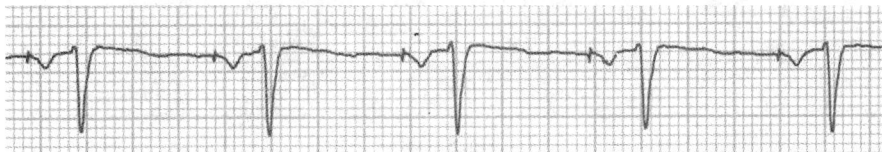

图5-43

（2）房室（A-V）顺序起搏，心室起搏（注意每个QRS前小的起搏信号）和心房感知正常窦性心律（注：起搏器信号有时很难看到）。

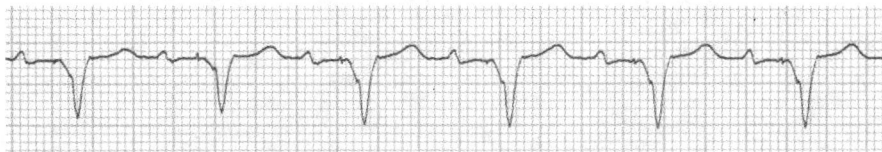

图5-44

（3）房室顺序起搏，既起搏心房也起搏心室（注意每个P波和QRS波前都有起搏信号）。

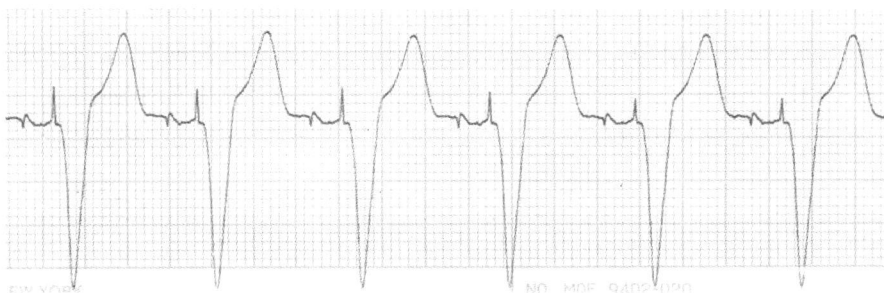

Fig. 5 – 45

（4）Normal functioning ventricular demand pacemaker. Small pacing spikes（arrows）are seen before QRS #1, #3, #4, and #6 representing the paced beats. There is marked sinus bradycardia（that's the reason for the pacemaker）, but when P waves are able to conduct they do（see QRS #2 and #5）. This is a nice example of incomplete AV dissociation due to sinus slowing where the artificial pacemaker takes over by default. Note also, in this V1 rhythm strip the morphology of the paced beats resemble QRS #2 in Fig. 5 – 25 indicative of a RV ectopic pacemaker focus（notched downstroke）.

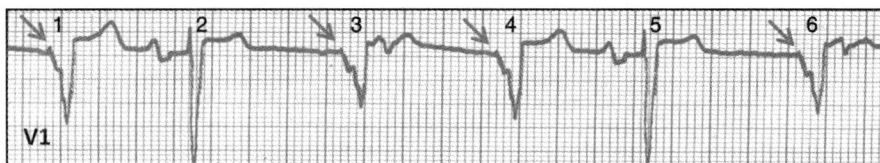

Fig. 5 – 46

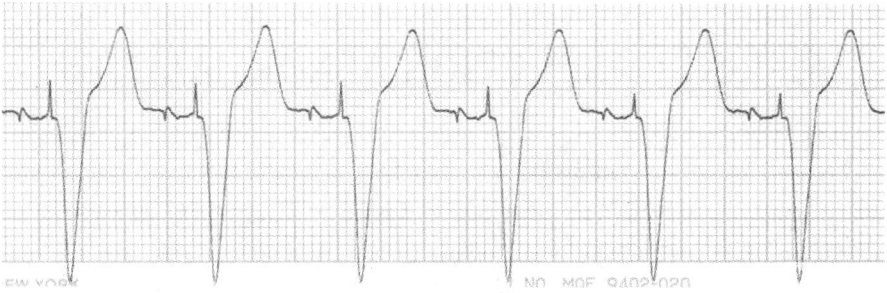

图 5 - 45

（4）正常功能的心室按需型起搏。QRS #1，#3，#4 和#6 前的小的起搏信号（箭头）是代表起搏心搏，有显著窦性心动过缓（植入起搏器的原因）。但当 P 波能够下传时，就自己进行夺获心室（见 QRS #2 和#5）。这是一个很好的例子，由于窦缓被人工起搏器默认接管导致的不完全的房室分离。还要注意，在这个 V1 导联中起搏的波形类似于图 5 - 25 中 QRS #2，表明这是一个右心室异位起搏点（下降支切迹），因为通常心室起搏电极都植入在右心室。

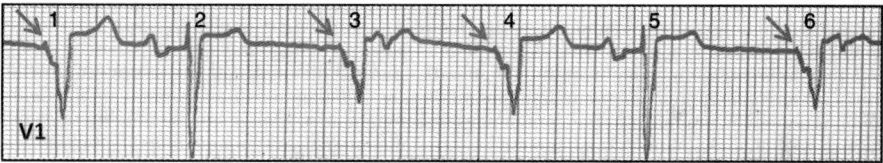

图 5 - 46

6 ECG CONDUCTION ABNORMALITIES

This section considers all disorders of impulse conduction that may occur within the cardiac conduction system (see diagram in Fig. 5 − 21). Heart block can occur anywhere in the specialized conduction system beginning with the sino-atrial connections, the AV junction, the bundle branches and fascicles, and ending in the distal ventricular Purkinje fibers. Disorders of conduction may manifest as slowed conduction (1st degree), intermittent conduction failure (2nd degree), or complete conduction failure (3rd degree). In addition, there are two varieties of 2nd degree heart block：Type I (or Wenckebach) (usually in the Ca^{2+} channel cells of the AV node) and Type II (or Mobitz) (usually in the Na^{+} channel cells of the bundle branches). In Type I (2nd degree) block decremental conduction is seen where the conduction velocity progressively slows beat-by-beat until failure of conduction occurs. This is the form of conduction block in the AV node. Type II block is all or noneand is more likely found in the His bundle or in the bundle branches and fascicles. The term exit block is used to identify a conduction delay or failure immediately distal to a pacemaker site. Sino-atrial (SA) block, for example, is an exit block. The following discussion considers conduction disorders in the anatomical sequence that defines the cardiac conduction system；so lets begin...

6.1 SINO-ATRIAL EXIT BLOCK (SA Block)：

6.1.1 2nd Degree SA Block

this is the only degree of SA block that can be recognized on the surface ECG (i. e. , an intermittent conduction failure between the sinus node and the right atrium). There are two types, although, because of sinus arrhythmia, they may be difficult to differentiate, and it is not clinically important to differentiate.

(1) Type I (SA Wenckebach)：the following 3 rules represent the classic rules of Wenckebach which were originally described for Type I 2nd degree AV block. The rules are the result of decremental conduction where the increment in conduction delay for each subsequent impulse gets smaller and smaller until conduction failure occurs. For Type I SA block the three rules are：

● PP intervals gradually shorten until a pause occurs (i. e. , the blocked sinus impulse fails to reach the atria；note, the sinus P-wave isn't seen on the ECG).

6　心电图传导异常

本章考虑可能发生在心脏传导系统所有的冲动传导障碍（见图5-21）。心脏传导阻滞可以发生在特定的传导系统的任何部位，无论从起始的窦房传导，房室结，束支及其分支，还是末端的心室传导的浦肯野纤维。传导障碍可能表现为缓慢传导（1度）、间歇传导异常（2度），或完全传导阻滞（3度）。此外，有两种类型的2度传导阻滞：Ⅰ型（或文氏型，通常在房室结的Ca^{2+}通道细胞）和Ⅱ型（或莫氏，通常在束支的Na^+通道细胞）。在2度Ⅰ型**递减传导阻滞**中，传导速度逐渐放缓直到传导不能发生，这是发生在房室结。2度Ⅱ型传导阻滞也称**全或无**的传导阻滞，多发生在希氏束或束支和浦肯野纤维。术语**传出阻滞**是用来识别一个传导延迟或在起搏点不能向远端传出。窦房阻滞（SAB）就是一个传出阻滞的例子。下面将讨论在解剖学上定义了的心脏传导系统的传导障碍……

6.1　窦房传出阻滞（窦房阻滞）

6.1.1　第2度窦房阻滞

2度窦房阻滞是唯一可以通过体表面心电图识别的窦房阻滞（例如在窦房结和右心房之间一个间歇性的传导阻断），其有两种类型，尽管如此，他们可能很难与窦性心律不齐区分，而且其鉴别的临床意义并不大。

（1）Ⅰ型（SAB文氏型）：正如在第2度Ⅰ型房室传导阻滞中所描述的，遵循经典的文氏的三原则。规则是递减传导的结果，每个后续的冲动传导延迟递增，心搏间距变得越来越小，直到传导中断。Ⅰ型窦房阻滞的三个规则是：

● PP间隔逐渐**缩短**直到产生间歇（即窦性冲动被阻滞不能传导到心房；注意，在心电图上是看不到窦房结冲动的）。

- The PP interval of the pause isless than the two preceding PP intervals.
- The PP interval following the pause (not seen on this ECG) is greater than the PP interval just before the pause.

Differential Diagnosis: marked sinus arrhythmia without SA block. The rhythm strip in Fig. 6 – 1 illustrates SA Wenckebach with a ladder diagram to show the progressive conduction delay between SA node and the atrial P wave. Note the similarity of this rhythm to marked sinus arrhythmia. Note also the timing between the SA firing and the atrial event (P wave) gets longer and longer until conduction failure occurs. Finally, the PP interval of the pause is less than the 2 preceding PP intervals.

Lead II

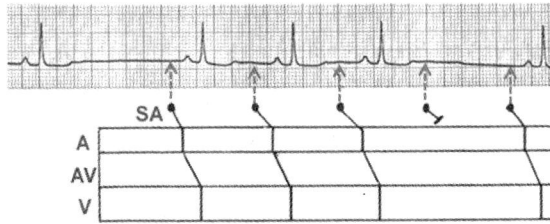

Sino-Atrial Exit Block (type)

Fig. 6 – 1

(2) Type II 2nd degree SA Block:

- PP intervals are fairly constant (unless sinus arrhythmia present) until conduction failure occurs.
- The pause is approximately twice the basic PP interval.

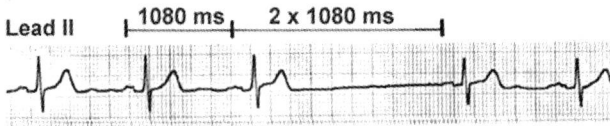

Lead II　1080 ms　2 x 1080 ms

Sino-Atrial Exit Block (Type II)

Fig. 6 – 2

- Both Type I and Type II SA block indicate sinus node disease (intrinsic or drug induced).

6.2 ATRIO-VENTRICULAR (AV) BLOCKS:

Possible sites of AV block:

- AV node (most common)
- His bundle (uncommon)

- 产生间歇的 PP 间隔小于其前面的 2 个 PP 间隔之和。
- 间歇后面的 PP 间隔（ECG 上没有显示）要**大于**间歇前面的 PP 间隔。

鉴别诊断：无窦房阻滞的显著的窦性心律不齐。下面的图 6 - 1 是用描述窦房文氏现象的梯形图来显示窦房结和心房 P 波之间的进展性传导延迟。注意这个节律与显著窦性心律不齐的相似性。还要注意从窦房结起搏到心房 P 波产生的时间越来越长，直到传导阻断。最后，暂停的 PP 间隔小于前面的 PP 间隔的 2 倍。

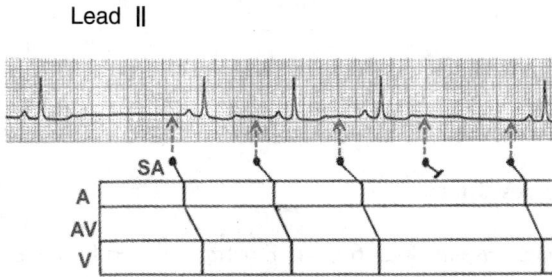

窦房传出阻滞（2 度 I 型）

图 6 - 1

（2）2 度 II 型窦房阻滞
- PP 间隔很稳定（除非存在窦性心律不齐）直到发生传导阻断（图 6 - 2）。

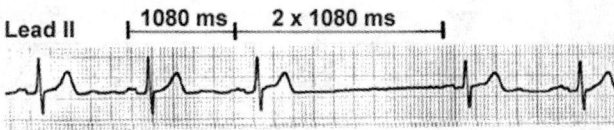

窦房传出阻滞（2 度 II 型）

图 6 - 2

- 产生的间歇大约相当于 2 倍的基本 PP 间隔。
- **无论 I 型还是 II 型窦房阻滞都提示窦房结病变（自身内在的或药物引起的）。**

6.2 房室传导阻滞（AVB）

房室阻滞的可能部位：
- 房室结（最常见的）
- 希氏束（少见）

● Bundle branch and fascicular divisions (in presence of already existing bundle branch block)

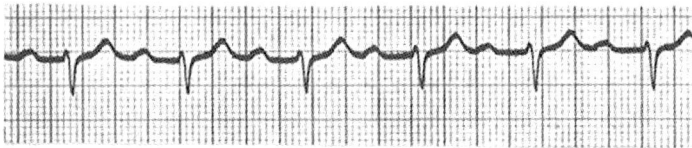

1 st degree AV block (PR = 280 ms)

Fig. 6 − 3

6.2.1 1st Degree AV Block

PR interval > 0.20 sec; all P waves conduct and are ollowed by QRS complexes.

6.2.2 2nd Degree AV Block

The ladder diagrams in Fig. 6 − 4 illustrate the differences between Type I (Wenckebach) and Type II 2nd degree AV block.

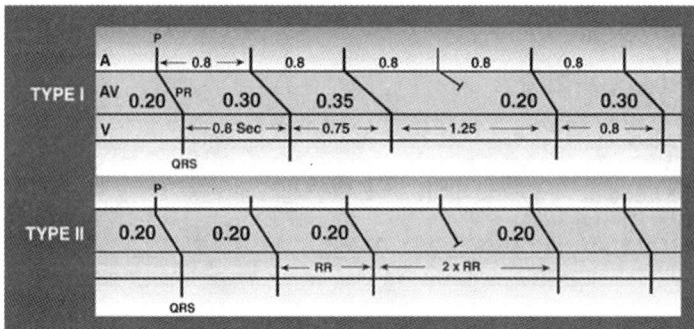

Fig. 6 − 4

(1) In "classic" Type I (Wenckebach) AV block the PR interval gets longer and longer (by smaller and smaller increments) until a nonconducted P wave occurs. The RR interval of the pause is less than the two preceding RR intervals, and the RR interval after the pause is greater than the RR interval just before the pause. These are the 3 classic rules of Wenckebach (described on P104 for the PP intervals in SA block). In Type II (Mobitz) AV block the PR intervals are constant (for at least 2 consecutive PR intervals) until a nonconducted P wave occurs. The RR interval of the pause is equal to the two preceding RR intervals (assuming a regular sinus rate). In 2 : 1 AV block one cannot distinguish type I from type II block (because PR is fixed in both cases). There are often other ECG clues to the correct diagnosis in 2 : 1 AV block:

● 束支及其分支(已经存在束支阻滞)

6.2.1 1度AVB

PR间期>0.20 s；所有P波都会跟随1个QRS波群。

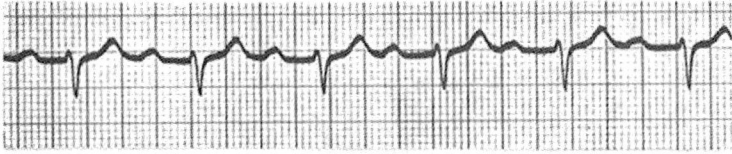

1度房室传导阻滞(PR = 280 ms)

图6-3

6.2.2 2度AVB

图6-4中的梯形图描述了Ⅰ型AVB(文氏型)与Ⅱ型AVB的区别。

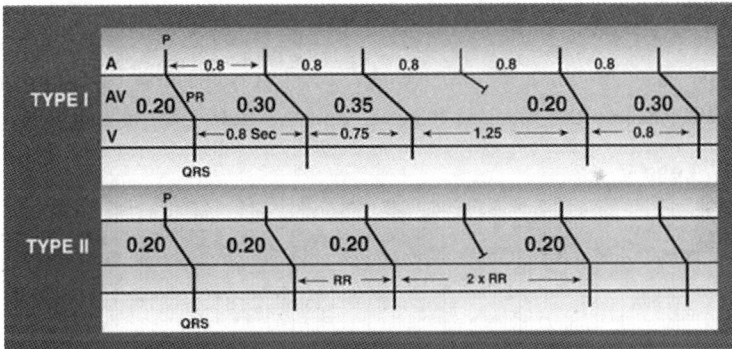

图6-4

(1)在"经典"Ⅰ型(文氏型)AVB中，PR间期越来越长(**通过叠加越来越小的增量**)，直到发生P不能下传。暂停的RR间隔小于前面两个RR间隔之和，并且暂停后的RR间隔大于暂停前的RR间隔。这些都是文氏现象的3个经典规则(P105中对窦房阻滞的PP间隔已有过描述)。Ⅱ型(莫氏)AVB的PP间隔是恒定的(至少2个连续的PR间期)，直到P不能下传发生。暂停的RR间隔等于前面的两个RR间隔之和(假设窦率是规律的)。在2:1的AVB中，无法区分Ⅰ型和Ⅱ型AVB(因为这两种情况下PR是固定的)时，要对2:1 AVB下正确的诊断经常需要有其他的心电图线索：

· Wide QRS complexes (BBB's) suggest type II; narrow QRS complexes suggest type I.

· Prolonged PR intervals (conducted beats) suggest type I (Wenckebach).

Lead V₁   "Classic Wenckebach"

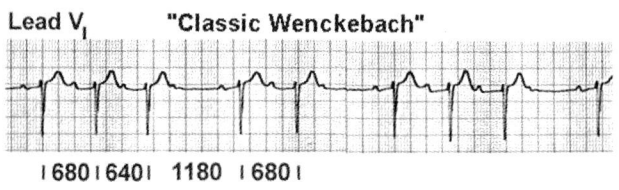

|680|640| 1180 |680|

Fig. 6 – 5

Type I (Wenckebach) 2nd degree AV block (note the RR intervals in ms duration illustrating the 3 classic rules):

NOTE: Type I AV block is almost always in the AV node itself, which means that the QRS duration is usually narrow, unless there is also a preexisting bundle branch block. Note also the 4:3 and 3:2 groupings of P's and QRS's. Group beating is common in type I 2nd degree AV block.

(2) Type II (Mobitz) 2nd degree AV block (note: the constant PR for two consecutive PR's before the blocked P wave, and the wide QRS of LBBB):

Lead V₁

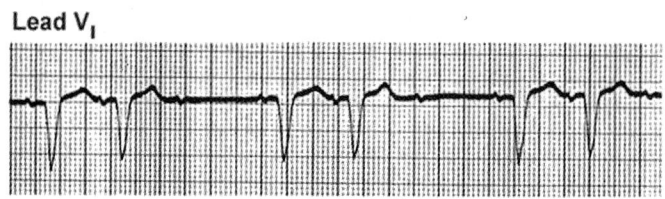

2nd degree AV block (type II) with LBBB

Fig. 6 – 6

Type II AV block there is almost always a preexisting bundle branch block (LBBB in the ECG strips above and below), which means that the QRS duration is wide indicating complete block of one bundle. The nonconducted P waves are blocked in the other bundle (i.e., a 2nd degree block in the right bundle branch). Also, in Type II block several consecutive P waves may be blocked as illustrated in Fig. 6 – 7:

Lead V₁

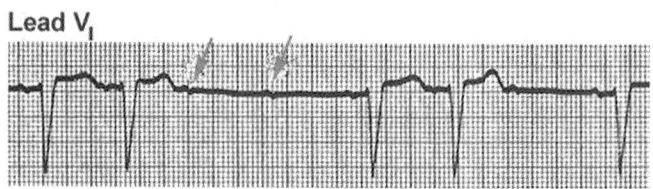

110

Fig. 6 – 7

- 宽 QRS 波群(BBB's)提示Ⅱ型 ABV；窄的 QRS 波群提示Ⅰ型 ABV。
- 延长的 PR 间期提示Ⅰ型 ABV(文氏型)。

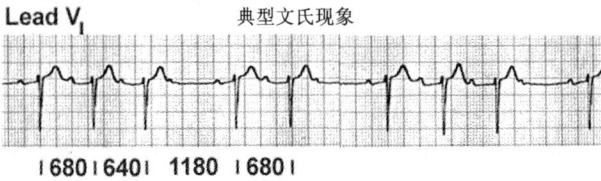

图 6-5

2 度Ⅰ型(文氏型)AVB(注意图 6-5 以毫秒为单位的 RR 间期说明经典的文氏三原则)。

注意：2 度Ⅰ型 AVB 几乎总是在房室结本身，这意味着 QRS 时限通常是窄的，除非还有一个先前存在的束支阻滞。还要注意 P 和 QRS 比例是 4:3 和 3:2 组合。这种组合往往是 2 度Ⅰ型 ABV 的方式传导阻滞。

(2)第 2 度Ⅱ型(莫氏型)AVB[见图 6-6，注意在 P 被阻断之前，两个连续的 PR 是一致的，而且是完全性左束支传导阻滞(LBBB)的宽的 QRS 波]

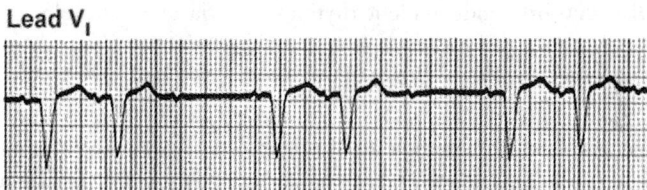

2 度Ⅱ型房室传导阻滞伴有左束支传导阻滞

图 6-6

2 度Ⅱ型 AVB 几乎总是有一个先前存在的束支阻滞(见上方和下方的心电图均有 LBBB)，这意味着 QRS 时限增宽就说明有 1 个束支已经阻滞了，P 不能下传说明另 1 个束支也阻滞了(即 2 度的右束支阻滞)。此外，2 度Ⅱ型阻滞可以连续几个 P 波被阻滞，如图 6-7 所示：

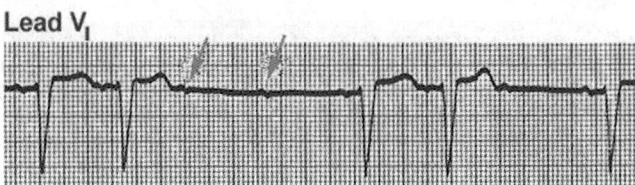

图 6-7

6.2.3 Complete (3rd Degree) AV Block

• Usually there iscomplete AV dissociation because the atria and ventricles are each controlled by independent pacemakers.

• Narrow QRS rhythms in 3rd degree AV block suggest a junctional escape focus indicating that the AV block is proximal to the bifurcation of the HIS bundle.

• Wide QRS rhythms suggest a ventricular escape focus (i. e. , often called an idioventricular rhythm). This is seen in ECG "A" below; ECG "B" shows the treatment for this 3rd degree AV

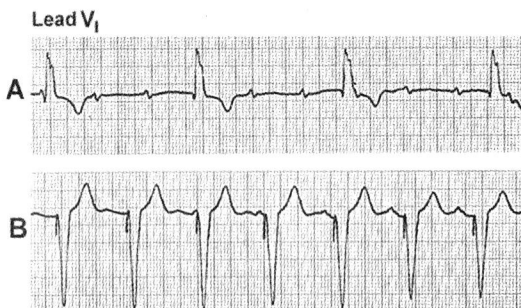

Fig. 6 – 8

block; i. e. , an artificialventricular pacemaker. The location of the block may be in the AV junction or bilaterally in the bundle branches. Look carefully in "B" for dissociated P waves that are independent of the pacemaker rhythm.

6.2.4 AV Dissociation (independent rhythms in atria and ventricles)

• Not synonymous with 3rd degree AV block, although AV block is one of the causes.

• May becomplete or incomplete. In complete AV dissociation the atria and ventricles are always independent of each other as seen in 3rd degree AV block. In incomplete AV dissociation there is either intermittent retrograde atrial capture from the ventricular focus or antegrade ventricular capture from the atrial focus.

• There arethree categories of AV dissociation (categories 1 & 2 are always incomplete AV dissociation):

(1) Slowing of the primary pacemaker (i. e. , SA node); a subsidiary escape pacemaker takes over by default. Note that in sinus arrhythmia two junctional beats take over when the sinus rate falls below the junctional escape rate.

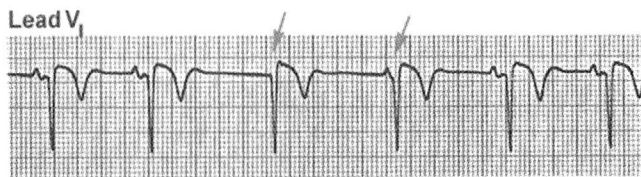

Incomplete AV dissociation due to sinus slowing (default) with junctional escapes (arrows)

Fig. 6 – 9

6.2.3 完全性(3度)AVB

● 通常有完全性的房室分离，是因为心房和心室被各自的起搏点控制。

● 3度AVB的QRS如果是窄的，提示交界区逸搏而且阻滞部位大约在希氏束的分支近端。

● 如果QRS是宽的，提示室性逸搏（即通常所指的**室性自主节律**），如下列心电图"A"；心电图"B"是经**人工心室起搏**治疗的3度AVB。阻滞部位可能在房室结或双束支。仔细看"B"中的分离P独立于起搏心律。

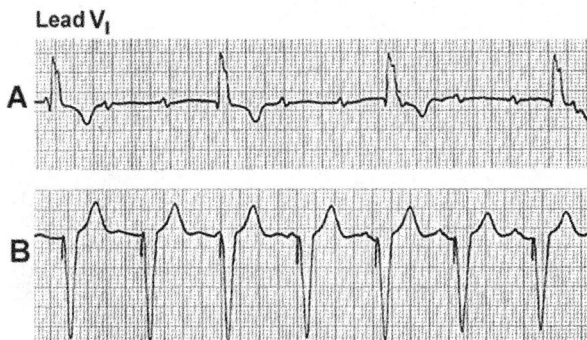

图6-8

6.2.4 房室分离(心房和心室各自独立)

● 房室分离和3度AVB不是同义词，尽管3度AVB是房室分离的许多原因之一。

● 房室分离可以是**完全性的或不完全性的**。完全性的房室分离心房和心室始终各自独立，正如3度AVB所见。不完全的房室分离可以一过性的由心室逆传心房并夺获心房，也可以由心房前传心室并夺获心室。

● 共有三种房室分离（第1和第2种是不完全的房室分离）：

（1）**原发的起搏点**（如窦房结）缓慢时，1个继发的逸搏起搏就会**取而代之**。注意在窦性心律不齐时，一旦窦性频率低于交界区频率，2个交界性逸搏就"上岗"了。

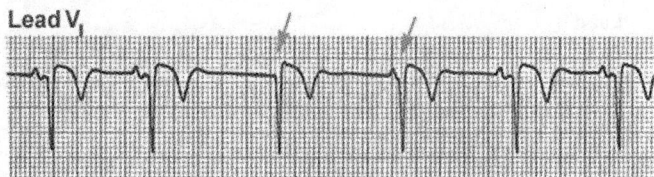

因窦性心动过缓导致不完全性房室分离伴交界性逸搏（箭头所示）

图6-9

（2）Acceleration of a subsidiary pacemaker that is slightly faster than the basic sinus rhythm; i. e. , take over by usurpation. In the example below 2 sinus beats are followed by an accelerated (or isochronic) ventricular rhythm (AVR). The first beat of the AVR takes over just before the 3rd sinus P wave would have conducted. During the AVR occasional sinus beats sneak into the ventricles and fusion beats may appear when the sinus beat and AVR beat merge in the ventricles.

Lead V$_1$

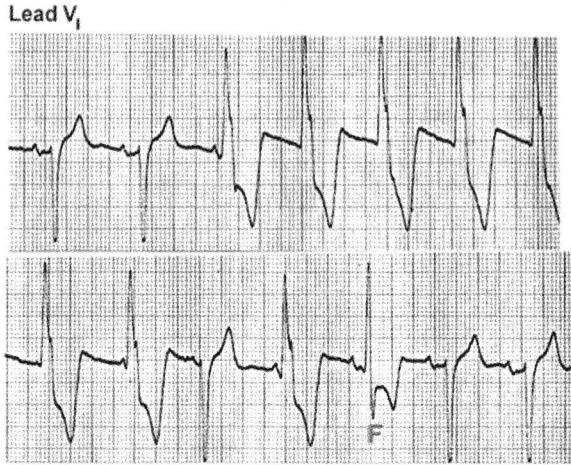

Incomplete AV dissociation (usurpation)

due to accelerated ventricular rhythm

F = fusion beat

Fig. 6 – 10

（3）2nd or 3rd degree AV block with an escape rhythm from a junctional site or a ventricular site：

• In the example (below) of complete AV dissociation (3rd degree AV bock with a junctional escape pacemaker) the PP intervals are alternating because of ventriculophasic sinus arrhythmia (phasic variations in vagal tone depending on the timing of ventricular contractions effect the sinus rate or PP intervals).

Lead II

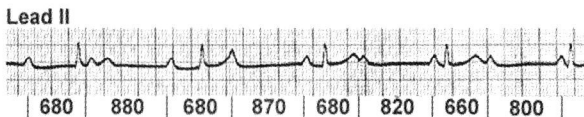

| 680 | 880 | 680 | 870 | 680 | 820 | 660 | 800 |

1. What is the diagnosis?

2. Why are the PP intervals alternating?

Fig. 6 – 11

(2)次级起搏点频率**加速**,只要略高于基本窦性心律,就会"抢班夺权"。在下面的例子中紧随2个窦性后的是一个加速的(或自主的)室性节律(AVR)。第一个室性心律波接管了第三个刚要下传的窦性P波。在室性节律中偶尔会有窦性节律潜入心室,当窦性节律和室性节律在心室相遇时可能会出现室性融合波。

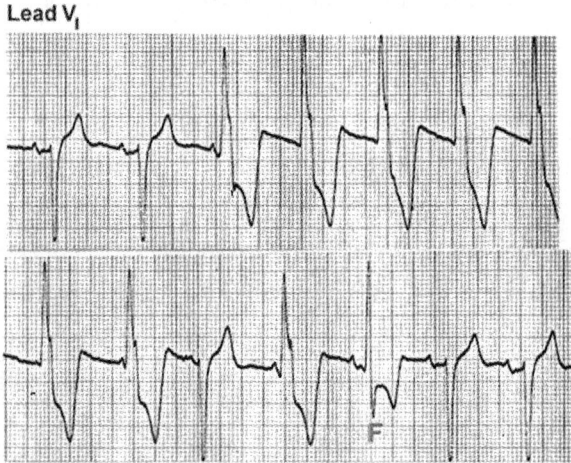

因加速性室性节律导致不完全性房室分离,F为融合波

图6-10

(3)**2度和3度AVB**伴有来自于1个交界区或心室起搏点的逸搏律:

图6-11是完全性房室分离的例子(3度AVB伴交界性逸搏律),PP间期的交互变化是由于**室相性窦性心律**不齐(迷走神经张力根据心室收缩时间对窦性频率或PP间期影响而发生时相变化)。也有另外一种观点认为长的PP间隔是由于窦房结缺血导致的。因为长的PP间隔内没有心室活动,窦房结灌注减少,机制同窦房结动脉或右冠病变引发的窦性心动过缓,而短的PP间隔内都有心室活动,窦房结得到正常灌注,P的出现没有延迟。

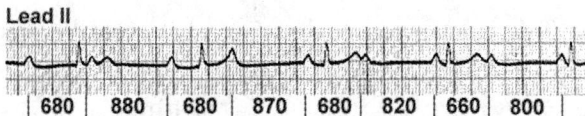

1. 诊断是什么?

2. 为什么PP间期发生交替性变化?

图6-11

6.3   INTRAVENTRICULAR BLOCKS

6.3.1   Right Bundle Branch Block (RBBB)

● "Complete" RBBB has a QRS duration $\geqslant 0.12$ s (120 ms)

● Close examination of QRS complex in various leads reveals that the terminal forces (i. e. , 2nd half of QRS) are oriented rightward and anterior because the right ventricle is depolarized after the left ventricle in RBBB.

· Terminal R′ wave in lead V1 (usually see rSR′ complex) indicating lateanterior forces.

· Terminal S waves in leads Ⅰ, aVL, V6 indicating laterightward forces.

· Terminal R wave in lead aVR also indicating laterightward forces.

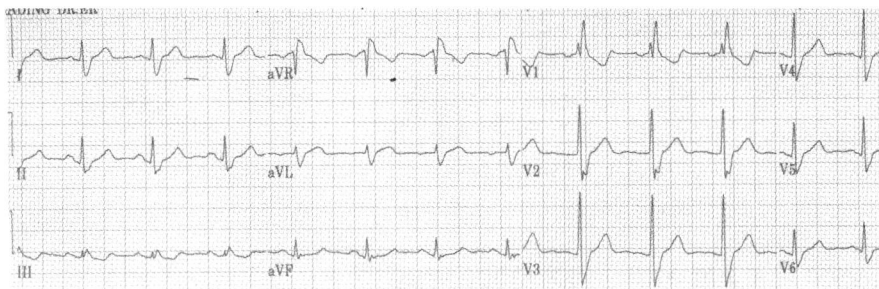

Fig. 6 – 12

● The frontal plane QRS axis in RBBB is usually in the normal range (i. e. , − 30 to +90 degrees). If left axis deviation is present, one must also considerleft anterior fascicular block, and if right axis deviation is present, one must consider left posterior fascicular block in addition to the RBBB (i. e. , bifascicular block).

● "Incomplete" RBBB has a QRS duration of 0.10 s − 0.12 s with the same 2nd half QRS features. This is often a normal variant, but could be seen in people with RVH.

● The "normal" ST – T wave morphology in RBBB is orientedopposite to the direction of the late QRS forces or last half of the QRS; i. e. , in leads with terminal R or R′ forces (e. g. , V1) the ST – T should be downwards (negative); in leads with late S forces (e. g. , Ⅰ, V6) the ST – T should be positive. If the ST – T waves are in the same direction as the terminal QRS forces, they should be labeled primary ST – T wave abnormalitiesbecause they may be related to other conditions affecting ST – T wave morphology (e. g. , ischemia, drug effects, electrolyte abnormalities).

6.3　心室内传导阻滞

6.3.1　右束支传导阻滞(RBBB)

- "完全性"RBBB 的 QRS 时间≥0.12 s(120 ms)。
- 仔细检查各导联的 QRS 波群发现其终末向量(即 QRS 波的后半部)是向右向前的,因为 RBBB 时右心室除极在左心室后。
  - V1 导联的终末 R′波(常见 rSR′波)指向较晚的**向前**向量。
  - Ⅰ,aVL,V6 导联的终末 S 波指向较晚的**向右**的向量。
  - aVR 导联的终末 R 波也指向较晚的**向右**的向量。

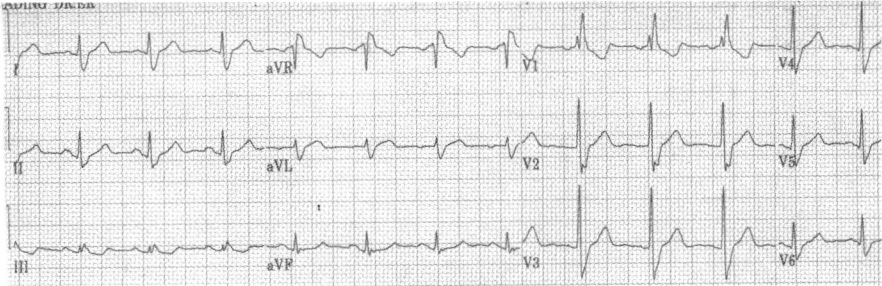

图 6 – 12

- RBBB 额面 QRS 电轴通常在正常范围(即 – 30°到 + 90°)。如果存在电轴左偏一定要考虑到左前分支阻滞(LAFB),如果电轴右偏一定要考虑到左后分支阻滞(LPFB),所以除考虑 RBBB 外,还要考虑分支阻滞。

- "不完全性"RBBB 的 QRS 时间为 0.10 ~ 0.12 s,QRS 波的后半部与完全性 RBBB 具有同样特征,这一点通常有正常变异,可见于右心室肥厚(RVH)的人。

- RBBB 的"正常"ST – T 波方向是与晚期 QRS 向量(QRS 后半部)相反的方向;也就是说,有终末 R 和 R′为主的导联(例如 V1)ST – T 应该向下(负向的);在后半部以 S 波为主的导联(如 V6)ST – T 应该是正向波。如果 ST – T 波与终末 QRS 主波向量方向一致,应该提示是**原发性 ST – T 波异常**,因为他们可能与其他影响 ST – T 波形态的状况有关(如缺血、药物影响、电解质异常)。

6.3.2 Left Bundle Branch Block (LBBB)

- "Complete" LBBB″ has a QRS duration ⩾0.12 s.

- Close examination of QRS complex (see ECG in Fig. 6 – 13) in various leads reveals that the terminal forces (i. e., 2nd half of QRS) are oriented leftward and posterior because the left ventricle is depolarized later after the right ventricle.

· Late S waves in lead V1 indicating lateposterior forces.

· Late R waves in lead Ⅰ, aVL, V6 indicating lateleftward forces.

· QRS complexes in leads Ⅰ, aVL, and V6 aremonophasic meaning that there should not be initial θ-waves or terminal S-waves in these leads (just wide R-waves with or without notches). The presence of θ-waves and/or S-waves in these leads may indicate scarred LV areas from old myocardial infarctions.

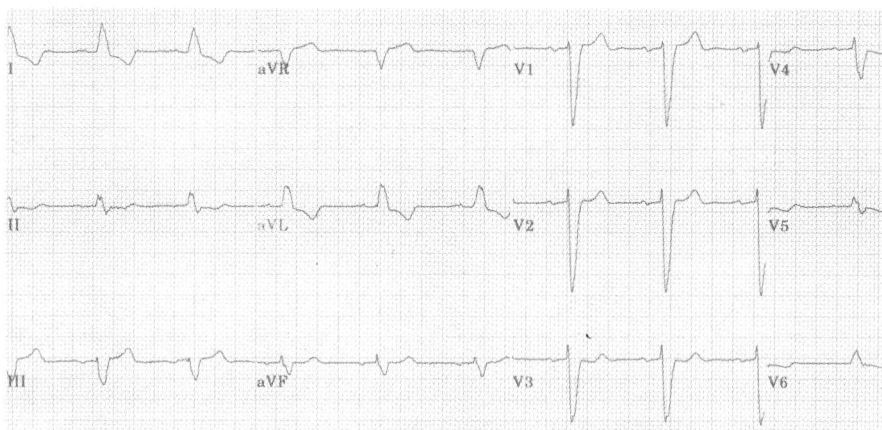

Fig. 6 – 13

- The "normal" ST – T waves in LBBB should be oriented opposite to the direction of the terminal QRS forces; i. e., in leads with terminal R or R′ forces the ST – T should be downwards (negative) (see Ⅰ, aVL); in leads with terminal S forces the ST – T should be upwards (positive) (see Ⅲ, V1 – V2). If the ST – T waves are in thesame direction as the terminal QRS forces, they should be labeled primary ST – T wave abnormalities. In the above ECG the ST – T waves are "normal" for LBBB; i. e., they are secondary to the change in the ventricular depolarization sequence.

- "Incomplete" LBBB looks like LBBB but QRS duration is 0.10 s – 0.12 s, with less ST – T change. This is often the result of long standing LVH.

6.3.2　左束支传导阻滞（LBBB）

● "完全性"LBBB 的 QRS 时间≥0.12 s。

● 仔细检查各导联的 QRS 波群（见图 6-13），揭示其终末向量（即 QRS 的后半部）都指向左和后，因为左心室除极在右心室之后。

·　V1 导联的后 S 波向量指向后面。

·　Ⅰ，aVL，V6 导联后 R 波向量指向左面。

·　Ⅰ，aVL，和 V6 的 QRS 波群单一型态意味着在这些导联没有起始 Q 波或终末 S 波（只是宽的 R 波伴或不伴有切迹）。如果这些导联存在 Q 波和/或 S 波提示左心室陈旧心肌梗死伴有瘢痕。

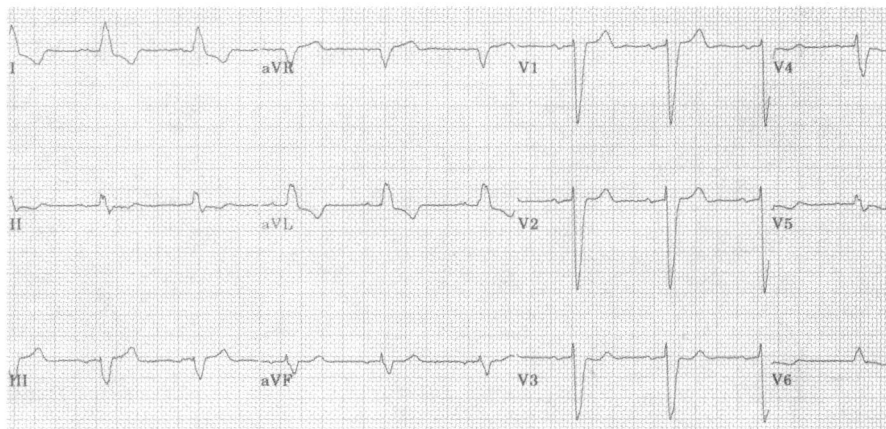

图 6-13

● "正常"LBBB 的 ST-T 波与终末 QRS 主波的方向相反；也就是说，在那些终末 R 和 R′为主波的导联，ST-T 应该向下（负向波）（见Ⅰ，aVL）；在终末 S 波为主的导联，ST-T 应该向上（正向波）（见 V1～V2，Ⅲ导联）。如果 ST-T 波与终末 QRS 主波在**相同方向**，应该表明是**原发性 ST-T 波异常**。在上面的心电图对 LBBB 来说 ST-T 波"正常"；也就是说，它们是**继发**于心室除极顺序的改变。

● "不完全"LBBB 看上去像完全性 LBBB，但 QRS 时限为 0.10～0.12 s，ST-T 改变更少，这通常是长期左心室肥厚（LVH）的结果。

6.3.3 Left Anterior Fascicular Block (LAFB)

—the most common intraventricular conduction defect

- Left axis deviation in frontal plane, usually −45 to −90 degrees
  - rS complexes in leads Ⅱ, Ⅲ, aVF (i. e., small initial r, large S)
  - S in Ⅲ > S in Ⅱ; R in aVL > R in aVR
  - Small q-wave in leads Iand/or aVL
  - R-peak time in lead aVL > 0.04 s, often with slurred R wave downstroke
  - QRS duration usually < 0.12 s unless coexisting RBBB
  - Usually see poor R progression in leads V1 – V3 and deeper S waves in leads
V5 and V6
  - Maymimic LVH voltage in lead aVL, and mask LVH voltage in leads V5, V6

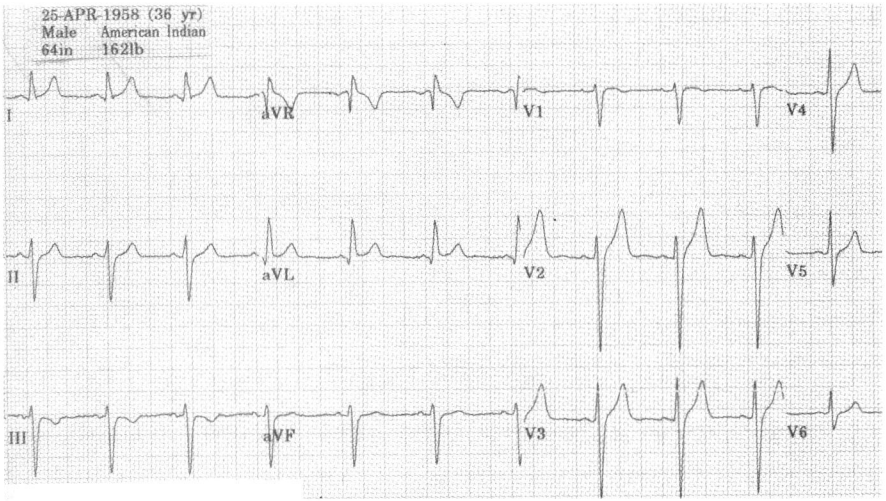

Fig. 6 – 14

In the above ECG, note −45° QRS axis, rS complexes in Ⅱ, Ⅲ, aVF, tiny q-wave in Ⅰ, aVL, S in Ⅲ > S in Ⅱ, R in aVL > R in aVR, and late S waves in leads V5 – 6. QRS duration is normal, and there is a slight slur to the R wave downstroke in lead aVL. This is classic LAFB!

6.3.3 左前分支阻滞(LAFB)——是最常见的室内传导缺陷

- 额面电轴左偏, 通常 −45°至 −90°。
- Ⅱ, Ⅲ, aVF 导联为 rS（即小 r, 大 S）。
- SⅢ > SⅡ; R aVL > R aVR。
- Ⅰ 和/或 aVL 导联小 q。
- aVL 导联 R 波达峰时间 >0.04 s, R 波降支通常有切迹。
- QRS 时间通常 <0.12 s, 除非同时存在 RBBB。
- 通常 V1~V3 导联 R 波发展的较差, 但是 V5~V6 导联的 S 波较深。
- 可能在 aVL 导联可模拟 LVH 电压, 但是在 V5, V6 可能掩盖 LVH 电压。

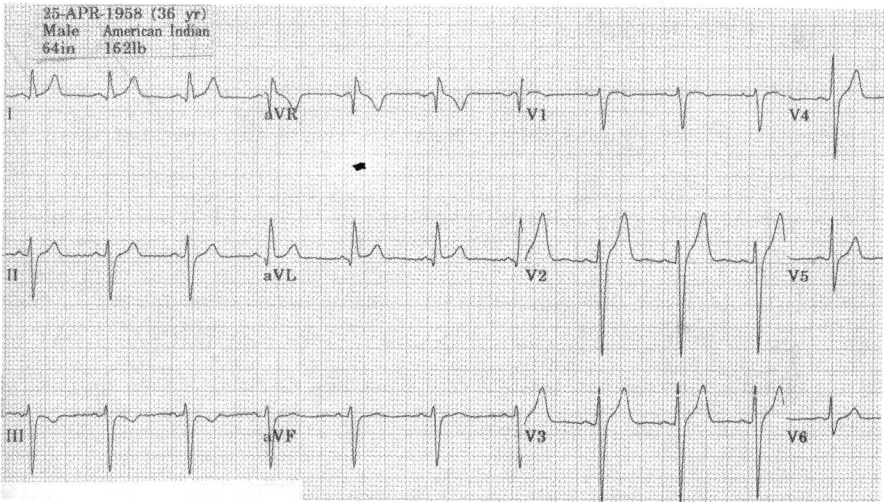

图 6 - 14

在图 6 - 14 的心电图中, 电轴 −45°, Ⅱ、Ⅲ、aVF 导联是 rS 波群, Ⅰ、aVL 导联小 q, SⅢ > SⅡ, R aVL > R aVR, S V5~V6。QRS 时间正常, 而且 aVL 导联 R 波降支有切迹, 这是**典型的 LAFB!**

6.3.4 Left Posterior Fascicular Block (LPFB)—Very rare intraventricular defect!

- Right axis deviation in the frontal plane (usually > +100°).

- rS complex in lead Ⅰ.

- qR complexes in leads Ⅱ, Ⅲ, aVF, with R in lead Ⅲ > R in lead Ⅱ.

- QRS duration usually <0.12 s unless coexisting RBBB.

- Must first exclude (on clinical information or imaging) other causes of right axis deviation such as cor pulmonale, pulmonary heart disease, pulmonary hypertension, etc., because these conditions or right heart strain can result in the identical ECG picture!

6.3.5 Bifascicular Blocks

- RBBB plus either LAFB (common) or LPFB (uncommon).

- Features of RBBB plus frontal plane features of the fascicular block (axis deviation, etc.)

- This ECG shows classic RBBB (note rSR′ in V1) plus LAFB (QRS axis = −60°, rS in Ⅱ, aVF; and small q in Ⅰ and aVL).

- Bifascicular blocks are clinically important precursors of complete (3rd degree) AV block. Before 3rd degree block occurs there may be episodes of 2nd degree AV block (Mobitz) indicating intermittent block in the remaining fascicle. These episodes often cause symptoms of syncope or presyncope.

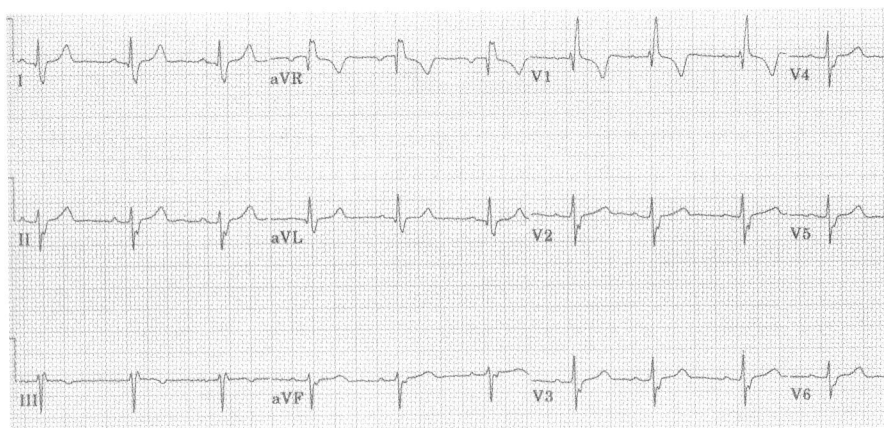

RBBB + LAFB (Bifascicular Block)

Fig. 6 – 15

6.3.4 左后分支阻滞(LPFB)——是非常罕见的室内传导缺陷!

- 额面电轴右偏(通常 > +100°)。
- Ⅰ 导联呈 rS 波群。
- Ⅱ,Ⅲ,aVF 导联为 qR 型,RⅢ > RⅡ。
- QRS 时间通常 <0.12 s,除非同时存在 RBBB。
- 必须首先除外(依据临床或影像信息)其他原因的电轴右偏,如肺心病,肺高压症等,因为这些情况或右心受累时可以有同样的心电图图像。

6.3.5 双分支阻滞

- RBBB 伴 LAFB(常见)或伴 LPFB(不常见)。
- RBBB 的特征加上分支阻滞的特征(额面电轴,等)。
- 这个 ECG 是典型的 RBBB(注意 V1 为 rSR′)加 LAFB(QRS 电轴 = -60°,Ⅱ,aVF 为 rS;而且 Ⅰ 和 aVL 为 q)。
- 双束支阻滞的临床重要性在于它是完全性(3 度)AVB 的先兆。在发生 3 度阻滞之前可能有数次的 2 度 AVB(莫氏)发作,提示剩余的分支存在间歇性阻滞。这些发作通常导致晕厥或黑矇(晕厥前状态)。

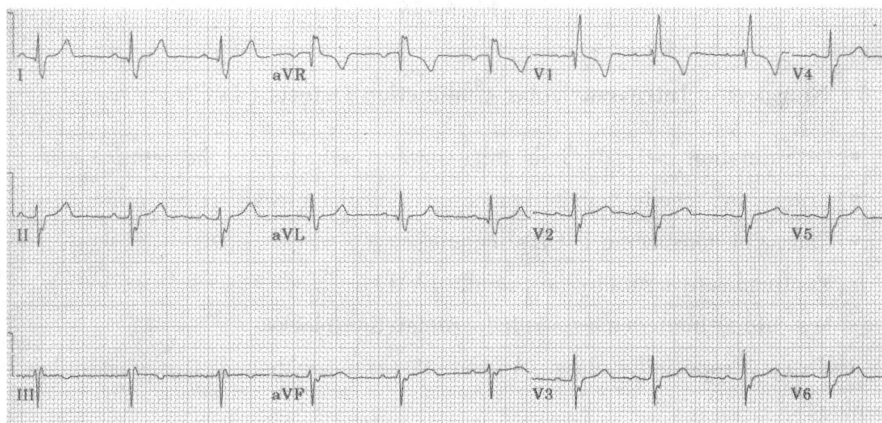

RBBB + LAFB(双分支阻滞:右束支传导阻滞 + 左前分支阻滞)

图 6 - 15

The ECG shown in Fig. 6 – 16 is classic RBBB and LPFB (bifascicular block) in a patient with chronic heart failure. Note the unusual frontal plane QRS axis of +150° (isoelectric lead Ⅱ), the rS complex in lead Ⅰ, and the small q-waves in Ⅱ, Ⅲ, aVF. There is rsR′ in V1 indicative of RBBB.

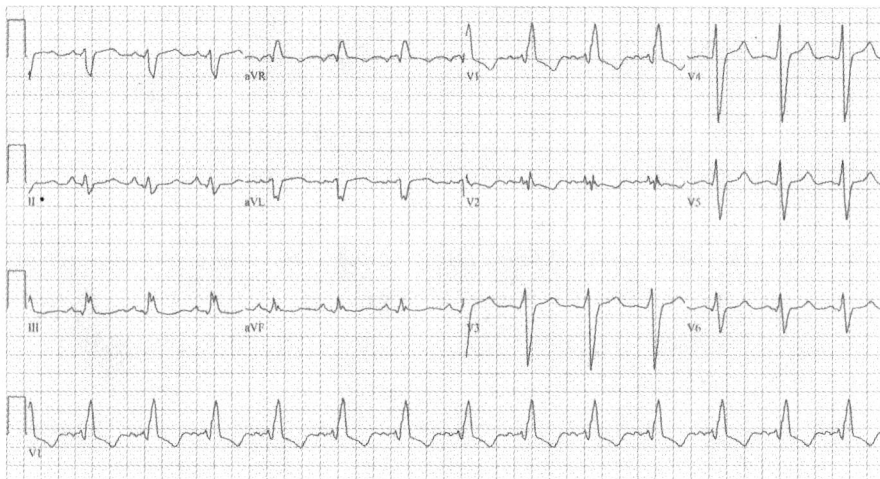

RBBB + LPFB (Bifascicular Block)

Fig. 6 – 16

6.3.6 Nonspecific Intraventricular Conduction Defects (IVCD)

- QRS duration > 0.10 s indicating slowed conduction in the ventricles.
- Criteria for specific bundle branch or fascicular blocks are not present.
- Causes of nonspecific IVCD's include：
- · Ventricular hypertrophy (especially LVH)
- · Myocardial infarction (so calledperiinfarction blocks)
- · Drugs, especially class IA and IC antiarrhythmics (e. g., quinidine, flecainide)
- · Severe hyperkalemia

图 6 – 16 的心电图是一个慢性心力衰竭患者的典型的 RBBB 伴 LPFB(双分支阻滞)。注意不寻常的 QRS 额面电轴 + 150°(等电位导联是 Ⅱ),Ⅰ 为 rS,Ⅱ,Ⅲ,aVF 为 q。V1 为 rSR′表明是 RBBB。

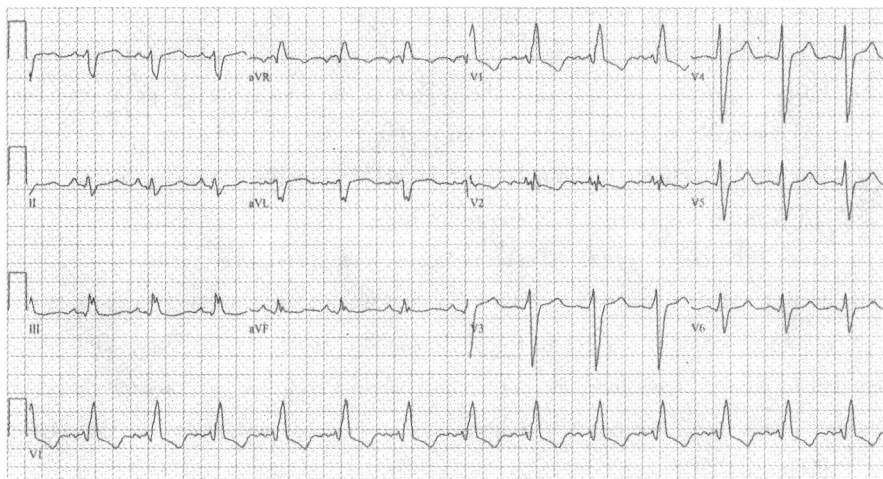

RBBB + LPFB(双分支阻滞:右束支传导阻滞 + 左后分支阻滞)

图 6 – 16

6.3.6 非特异性室内传导缺陷(IVCD)

- QRS 时间 >0.10 s 表明室内传导减慢。
- 不存在特异性束支和分支阻滞的标准。
- **非特异性** IVCD's 原因包括:
- · 心室肥大(尤其是 LVH)
- · 心肌梗死(所谓**梗死周围阻滞**)
- · 药物,尤其是 IA 和 IC 类抗心律失常药(如奎尼丁,氟卡尼)
- · 严重的高钾血症

6.4 Wolff-Parkinson-White (WPW) Preexcitation

Although not a true IVCD, this condition causes widening of QRS complex and, therefore, deserves to be considered here)

(1) The QRS complex represents afusion between two ventricular activation fronts:

· Early ventricular activation in the region of the accessory AV pathway (Bundle of Kent). This is illustrated in the diagram in Fig. 4 – 1.

· Ventricular activation through the normal AV junction, bundle branch system.

(2) ECG criteria include all of the following:

· Short PR interval (<0.12 s) due to early ventricular activation

· Initial slurring of QRS complex (delta wave) representing early ventricular activation into ventricular muscle in the region of the accessory pathway. Delta waves, if negative in polarity (see lead Ⅲ, aVF, and V1 in Fig. 6 – 17), may mimic infarct Q waves and result in a false positive diagnosis of myocardial infarction.

· Prolonged QRS duration (usually >0.10 s)

· Secondary ST – T changes due to the altered ventricular activation sequence

· QRS morphology, including polarity of delta wave depends on the particular location of the accessory pathway as well as on the relative proportion of the QRS complex that is due to early ventricular activation (i. e. , degree of fusion).

· The accessory pathway enables episodes of PSVT to occur (circus rhythm).

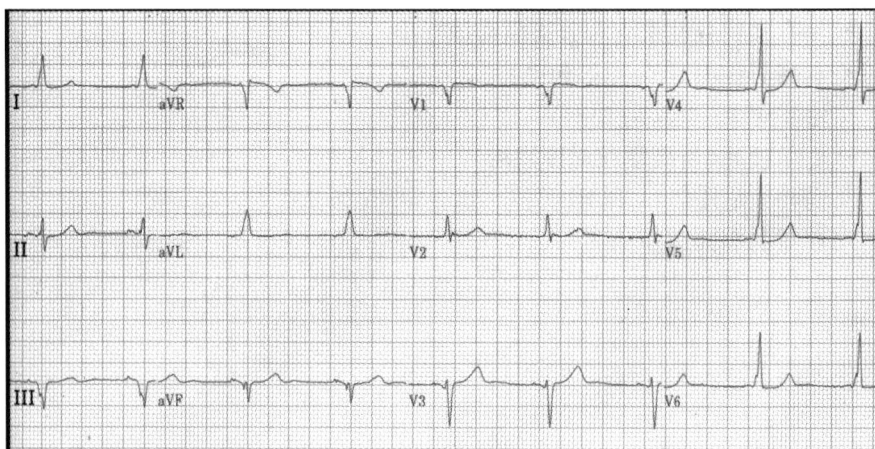

WPW Preexcitation (note short PR and delta waves best seen in Ⅰ, V5 – V6)

Fig. 6 – 17

6.4 预激综合征(WPW)

尽管不是真正的室内传导缺陷(IVCD),但是这种情况也导致宽大的 QRS 波群,因此,值得在此一并讨论。

(1)这个宽的 QRS 波群是**两部分心室兴奋的融合**:

● 较早的兴奋的部分心室是房室旁路(**Kent's 束**)的部位。见图 4 – 1 的图示说明。

● 另一部分心室兴奋是通过正常的房室结,束支系统传导的。

(2)心电图标准包括下列所有条件:

● 短 PR 间期(< 0. 12 s),由于心室提前兴奋所致 QRS 初始的黏合波(**delta 波**)代表旁路部位心室肌的早期兴奋。

● 如果 delta 波的极性是负的(见图 6 – 17 中的Ⅲ,aVF 和 V1 导联),很可能模拟梗死 Q 波并导致心肌梗死的假阳性诊断。

● QRS 时间(通常 > 0. 10 s)。

● 继发性 ST – T 改变与心室兴奋顺序改变有关。

● QRS 形态,包括 delta 波的极性取决于旁路特定位置和早期兴奋在 QRS 波群中所占的相对比例(即融合程度)。

● 旁路也可导致室上性心动过速(PSVT)发作(折返节律)。

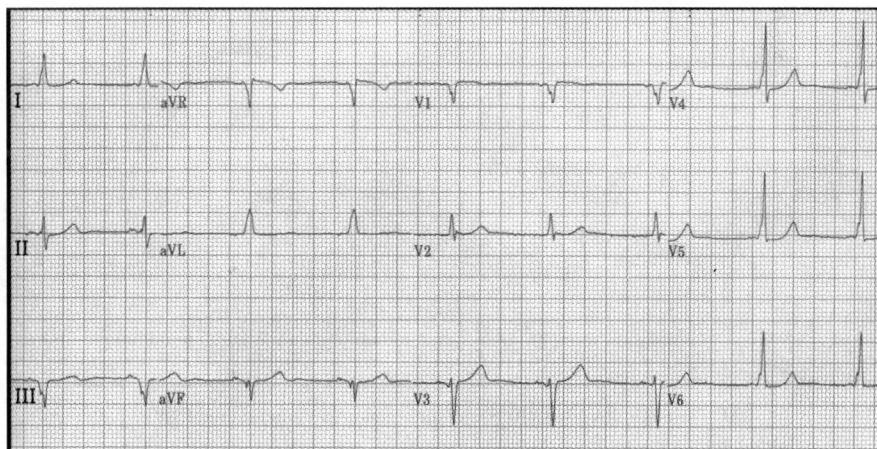

预激综合征(注意短 PR 和 delta 波在Ⅰ,V5 ~ V6 导联最明显)

图 6 – 17

7　ATRIAL ENLARGEMENT

7.1　**Right Atrial Enlargement**（RAE，P-pulmonale，"Viagra P-waves"）

- P wave amplitude >2.5 mm in Ⅱ and/or >1.5 mm in V1（these criteria are not very specific or sensitive）
- Frontal plane P-wave axis≥90°（isoelectric in lead I）
- Better criteria can be derived from the QRS complex; these QRS changes are due to both the high incidence of RVH when RAE is present, and the RV displacement by an enlarged right atrium.

  · QR, Qr, qR, or qRs morphology in lead V1（in absence of coronary heart disease）

  · QRS voltage in V1 is <5 mmand V2/V1 voltage ratio is >6（Sensitivity = 50%; Specificity =90%）

  · Why are these P waves（see lead Ⅱ below）sometimes called "Viagra P-waves"?

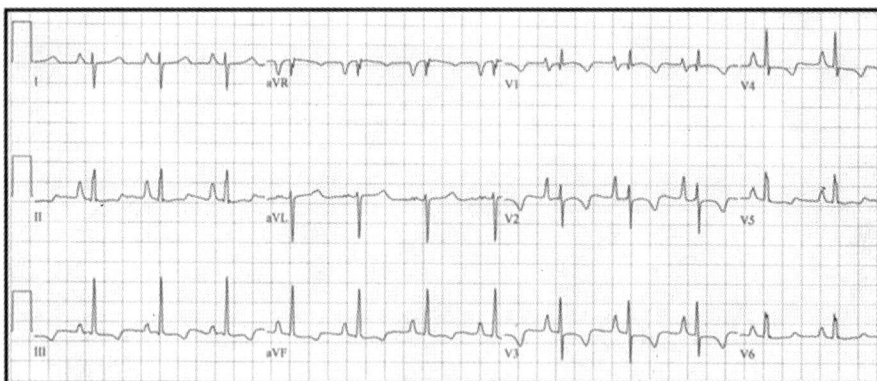

RAE：note also RAD（+110°）and qR complex in V1 indicative of RVH

Fig. 7－1

7.2　**Left Atrial Enlargement**（**LAE，** P-mitrale）

- P wave duration≥0.12 s in frontal plane（usually lead Ⅱ）
- Notched P wave in limb leads with interpeak duration ≥0.04 s

7 心房增大

7.1 右心房增大（肺性 P 波，"伟哥 P 波"）

• Ⅱ 导联 P 振幅 >2.5 mm 和/或 V1 导联 >1.5 mm（这些标准既不特异又不敏感）。

• 额面 P 波电轴 ≥90°（Ⅰ 导联是等电导联）。

• 较好的标准来自于 QRS 波群；这些 QRS 改变来自于只要有右心房大就会有右心室大的高发生率。

· V1 导联可见 QR，Qr，qR 或 qRs 形态（冠心病除外）。

· V1 导联 QRS 电压 <5 mV 而且 V2/V1 电压 >6（敏感性 =50%；特异性 =90%）。

· 为什么这些 P 波（见下面 Ⅱ 导联）有时被称为"伟哥 P 波"？!

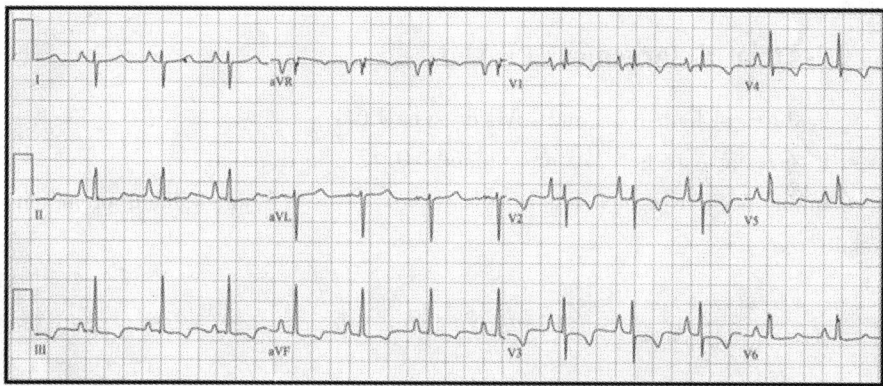

RAE：还要注意电轴右偏（+110°）以及 V1 导联为 qR 波群提示是右心室肥大（RVH）。

图 7-1

7.2 左心房增大（LAE，二尖瓣 P）

• P 波时间 ≥0.12 s（额面，通常以 Ⅱ 导联为准）。

• 肢体导联 P 波可见切迹，切迹两侧峰间距 ≥0.04 s。

● Terminal P negativity in lead V1（i. e. ,"P-terminal force"）duration $\geqslant 0.04$ s, depth $\geqslant 1$ mm.

● Sensitivity $=50\%$; Specificity $=90\%$

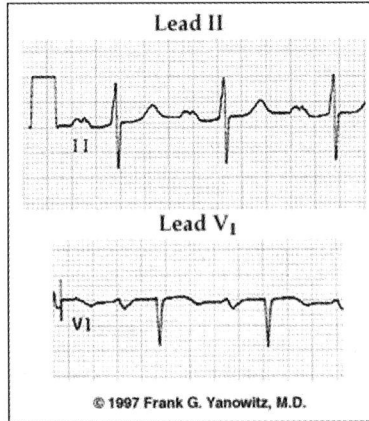

Classic LAE in lead Ⅱ and V1（with 1st degree AV block）

Fig. 7 −2

7.3   Bi-Atrial Enlargement（BAE）

● Features of both RAE and LAE in same ECG

● P wave in lead Ⅱ >2.5 mm talland >0.12 s in duration

● Initial positive component of P wave in V1 >1.5 mm talland prominent P-terminal force

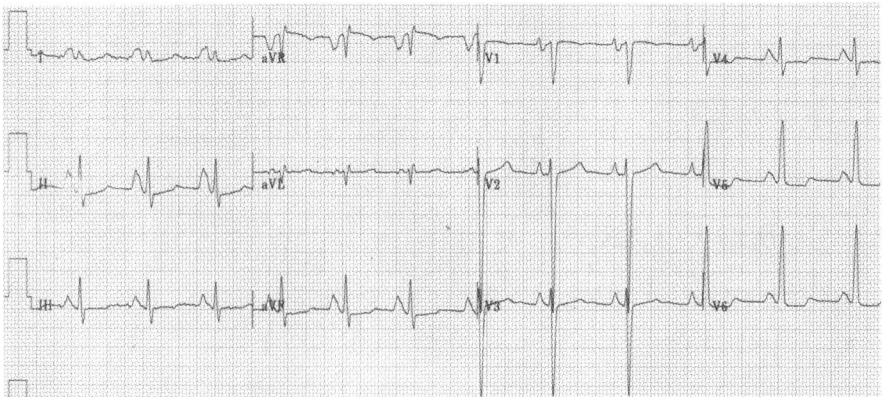

Bi-Atrial Enlargement with LVH

Fig. 7 −3

- V1 导联终末 P 为负向波（即"终末 P 为主"）时间≥0.04 s，深度≥1 mm。
- 敏感性 = 50%；特异性 = 90%。

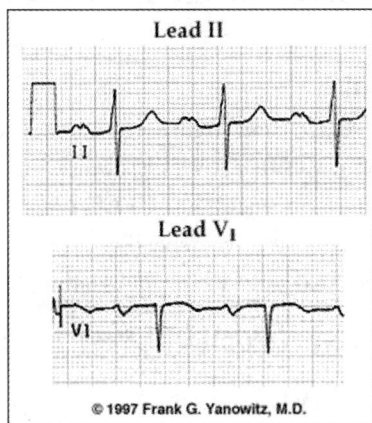

典型的左心房大表现在Ⅱ和 V1 导联（伴 1 度 AVB）

图 7 - 2

7.3 双心房增大（BAE）

- 在同一心电图中既有右心房大又有左心房大的特征。
- Ⅱ P 波高度 > 2.5 mm 而且时间 > 0.12 s。
- V1 P 波的初始成分是正向高度 > 1.5 mm，而且终末 P 成分为负向并以负向为主。

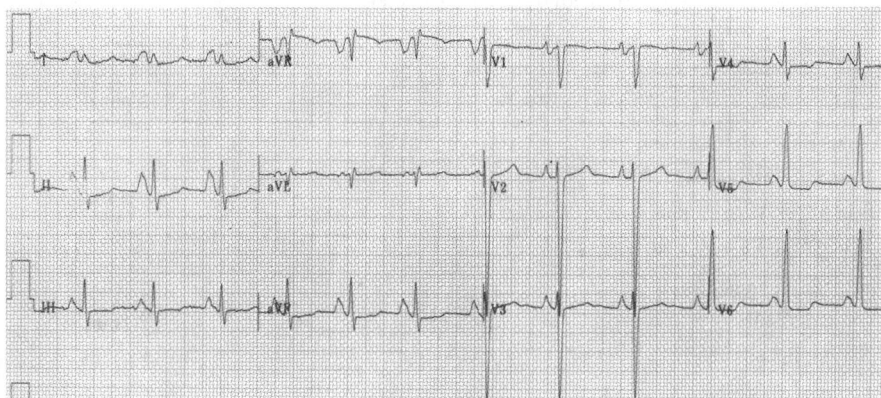

双房增大伴左心室大（LVH）

图 7 - 3

8   VENTRICULAR HYPERTROPHY

Introductory Information：

The ECG criteria for diagnosing right or left ventricular hypertrophy arevery insensitive (i. e. , sensitivity ~ 50% , which means that ~ 50% of patients with ventricular hypertrophy cannot be recognized by ECG criteria). When in doubt... Get an ECHO! However, the criteria are very specific (i. e. , specificity > 90% , which means if the criteria are met, it is very likely that ventricular hypertrophy is present).

8.1   Left Ventricular Hypertrophy (LVH)

（1）General ECG features include：

• QRS amplitude：voltage criteria；i. e. , tall R-waves inLV leads (Ⅰ , aVL, V5 – 6), deep S-waves in RV leads (V1 – 3).

• Delayedintrinsicoid deflection in V5 or V6 (i. e. , the time from QRS onset to peak R is ≥0. 05 sec)

• Widened QRS/T angle (i. e. , left ventricular strain pattern or ST – T waves oriented opposite to QRS direction). This pattern is more common with LVH due to pressure overload (e. g. , aortic stenosis, systemic hypertension) rather than volume overload.

• Leftward shift in frontal plane QRS axis (not necessarily in LAD territory)

• Evidence forleft atrial enlargement (LAE)

Table 8 – 1   ROMHILT-ESTES Criteria for LVH ("definite" ≥5 points；"probable" 4 points)

+ ECG Criteria	Points
Voltage Criteria (any of)： R or S in limb leads≥20 mm S in V1 or V2≥30 mm R in V5 or V6≥30 mm	3 points
ST – T Abnormalities： On digitalis Rx Not on digitalis Rx	1 point 3 points
Left Atrial Enlargement in V1	3 points
Left axis deviation≥ – 30°	2 points
QRS duration≥0. 09 sec	1 point
Delayed intrinsicoid deflection in V5 or V6 (≥0.05 sec)	1 point

8　心室肥大

基本信息介绍：

心电图诊断右或左心室肥大的标准非常不敏感（即灵敏度大约 50%，这意味着约有 50% 的患者的心室肥大不能通过心电图的标准来识别）。如果有疑问，去做超声！然而心电图的标准具有很好的特异性（例如特异性 > 90%，这意味着如果条件得到满足，则很可能存在心室肥大）。

8.1　左心室肥大（LVH）

一般的心电图特征包括：

● QRS 振幅：电压标准；即左心导联（Ⅰ，aVL，V5 ~ V6）高的 R 波，右心导联（V1 ~ V3）深的 S 波。

● V5 或 V6 导联的**室壁激动时间（intrinsicoid deflection）**延长（即从 QRS 起始到达 R 波顶峰的时间 ≥ 0.05 s）。

● QRS/T 夹角增宽（即左心室压力模式，ST – T 朝向与 QRS 方向相反）。该模式在压力过负荷导致的左心室肥厚较容量过负荷更为常见（如主动脉狭窄，系统性高血压）。

● 额面 QRS 电轴向左（但不一定在电轴左偏的范围内）。

● 左心房大（LAE）的证据。

表 8 – 1　ROMHILT-ESTES 左心室大的计分标准（"确切" ≥ 5 分；"可疑" 4 分）

心电图标准	计分标准（分）
电压标准（任何 1 项）： 肢体导联 R 或 S ≥ 20 mm S V1 或 V2 ≥ 30 mm R V5 或 V6 ≥ 30 mm	3
ST – T 改变： 应用地高辛 未用地高辛	1 3
V1 导联为左心房大	3
电轴左偏 ≥ – 30°	2
QRS 时间 ≥ 0.09 s	1
V5 或 V6 室壁激动时间延长 ≥ 0.05 s	1

（2）CORNELL Voltage Criteria for LVH（sensitivity = 22%, specificity = 95%）：

- S in V3 + R in aVL > 28 mm（men）
- S in V3 + R in aVL > 20 mm（women）

（3）Other Voltage Criteria for LVH（note that voltage criteria alone can't make a "definite" ECG diagnosis of LVH）

- Limb-lead voltage criteria：
- · R in aVL ≥ 11 mm or, if left axis deviation, R in aVL ≥ 18 mm
- · R in I + S in Ⅲ > 25 mm
- · R in aVF > 20 mm
- · S in aVR > 14 mm
- Chest-lead voltage criteria：
- · S in V1 + R in V5 or V6 ≥ 35 mm
- · R + S in any leads > 45 mm

Example 1：Limb-lead Voltage Criteria; e. g., R in aVL > 11 mm, or R in I + S in Ⅲ > 25 mm; note downsloping ST segment depression in leads Ⅰ and aVL.）

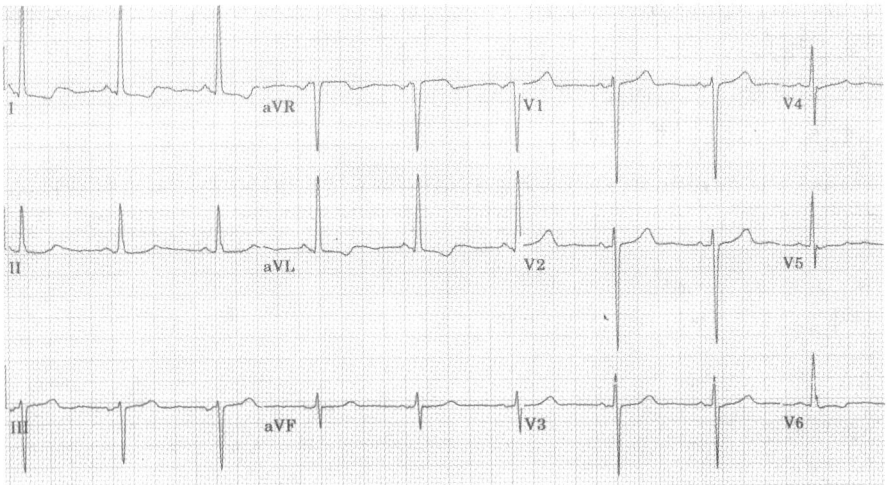

Fig. 8 − 1

(2)康奈尔(CORNELL) LVH 电压标准（敏感性 =22%，特异性 =95%）。

- S V3 + R aVL > 28 mm(男性)。
- S V3 + R aVL > 20 mm(女性)。

(3)LVH 的其他电压标准(注意单凭电压标准不能"确定"左心室肥厚的心电图诊断)

- 肢体导联电压标准：
- · R aVL≥11 mm，或如果电轴左偏，R aVL≥18 mm。
- · R I + S Ⅲ > 25 mm。
- · R aVF > 20 mm。
- · S aVR > 14 mm。
- 胸导联电压标准：
- · S V1 + R V5 或 V6≥35 mm。
- · 任何导联 R + S > 45 mm。

例1：肢体导联电压标准，即 R aVL > 11 mm，或 R I + S Ⅲ > 25 mm；注意 I 和 aVL 导联的 ST 段斜形向下压低。

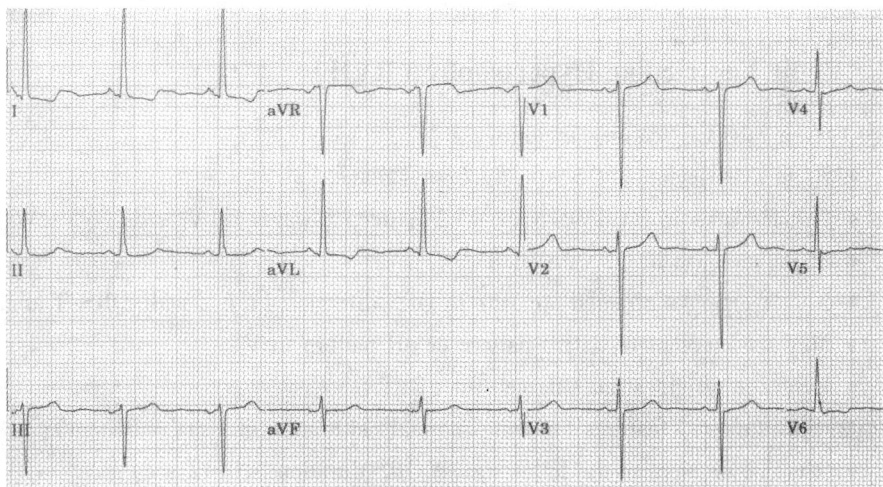

图 8 - 1

Example 2：ROMHILT-ESTES Criteria：3 points for precordial lead voltage，3 points for ST – T changes；also LAE（possibly bi-atrial enlargement）. This pattern is classic for LVH due to severe LV pressure overload as seen in aortic stenosis.

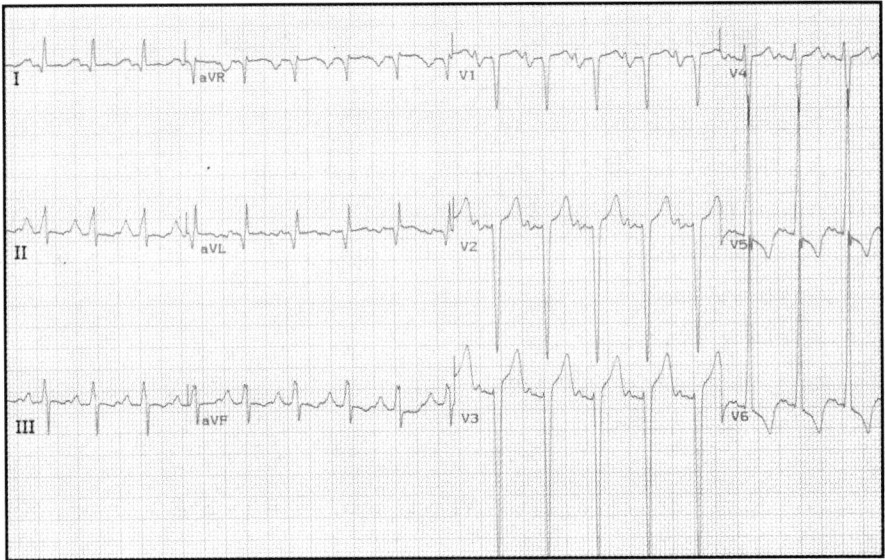

Fig. 8 – 2

8.2 Right Ventricular Hypertrophy（RVH）

（1）General ECG features include：

- Right axis deviation（>90°）in frontal plane
- Tall R-waves in RV leads（V1 – V2）；deep S-waves inLV leads（V5 – V6）
- Slight increase in QRS duration
- ST – T changes directed opposite to QRS direction（i. e. , wide QRS/T angle）
- May see incomplete RBBB pattern or qR pattern in V1
- Evidence ofright atrial enlargement（RAE）

（2）Specific ECG features（assumes normal calibration of 1 mV = 10 mm）：

- Any one or more of the following（if QRS duration <0. 12 sec）：

· Right axis deviation（>90 degrees）in presence of disease capable of causing RVH

　　· R in aVR >5 mm, or

　　· R in aVR > Q in aVR

例 2：ROMHILT-ESTES 评分标准：胸导联电压 3 分，ST - T 改变 3 分；还有左心房大（LAE）（可能双房大）也是 3 分。这一模式是左心室大的经典模式，见于主动脉狭窄所致的严重的左心室压力超负荷。

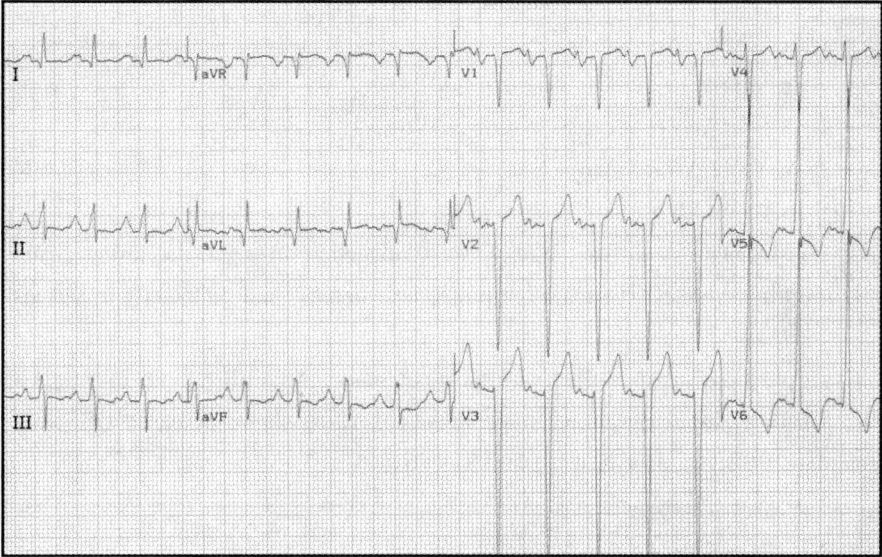

图 8 - 2

8.2 右心室肥大（RVH）

（1）一般的心电图特征包括：

- 额面电轴右偏（>90°）。
- 右心室导联（V1 - V2）R 波较高；左心室导联（V5 - V6）S 波较深。
- QRS 时间轻微增加。
- ST - T 改变与 QRS 方向相反（如宽大的 QRS/T 夹角）。
- V1 导联可以见到不完全的 RBBB 或 qR 波形。
- 右心房大（RAE）的证据。

（2）特异的 ECG 特征（如果正常标定 1 mV = 10 mm）：

- 具有下列之一或以上者（如果 QRS 时间 <0.12 s）：
- 电轴右偏（>90°）并存在可能导致右心室大的疾病。
- R aVR >5 mm，或
- R aVR > Q aVR

- Any one of the following in lead V1:
- · R/S ratio > 1 and negative T wave
- · qR pattern (see Example 1 in Fig. 8 – 3)
- · R > 7 mm, or S < 2mm, or rSR′ with R′ > 10 mm
- Other chest lead criteria:
- · R in V1 + S in V5 (or V6) 10 mm
- · R/S ratio in V1 > 1 or S/R ratio in V6 > 1
- · R in V5 or V6 < 5 mm
- · S in V5 or V6 > 7 mm
- ST segment depression and T wave inversion in right precordial leads are usually seen in severe RVH such as in pulmonary stenosis and pulmonary hypertension.

Example 1: RVH in patient with mitral stenosis. Note qR pattern in V1, marked RAD (+ 140°), large P-terminal force in V1 (LAE), slight increased QRS duration (incomplete RBBB), deep S wave in V5 – V6.

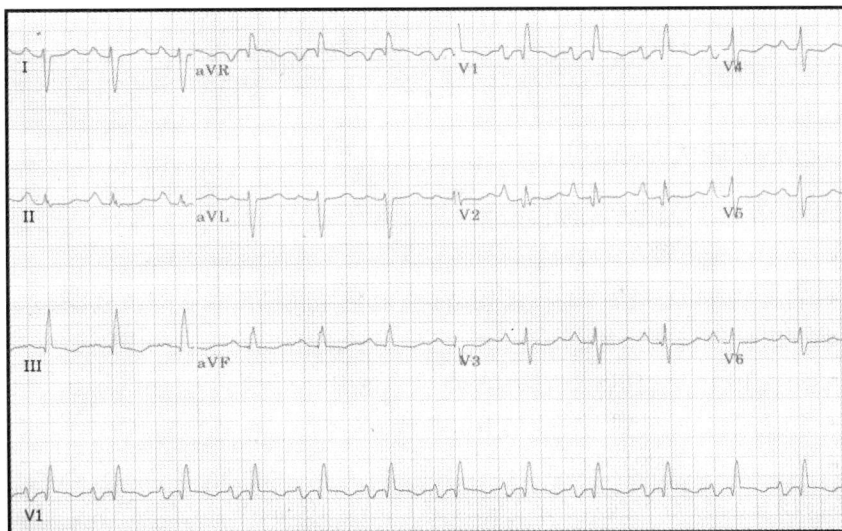

Fig. 8 – 3

Example 2: 18 yr. old patient with primary pulmonary hypertension. Note: marked RAD (+ 140°), R in V1 > 7mm, prominent anterior forces in V1 – V3, increased P amplitude of RAE, and the typical RV strain pattern in precordial leads (ST depression, T wave inversion).

- V1 导联有下列任何 1 项：
· R/S > 1 而且 T 波是负向波。
· qR 型（见图 8 – 3 中例子 1）。
· R > 7 mm，或 S < 2mm，或 rSR′的 R′> 10 mm。
- 其他胸导联标准：
· R V1 + S V5（或 6）≥10 mm。
· R/S V1 >1 或 V6 的 S/R >1。
· R V5 或 V6 <5 mm。
· S V5 或 V6 >7 mm。
- 严重的右心室肥大常见 ST 段压低和 T 波倒置，如肺动脉狭窄和肺动脉高压。

例1：患有二尖瓣狭窄的 RVH 患者。注意 V1 是 qR 型，明显电轴右偏（ +140°），V1 较大的终末 P 为主（LAE），QRS 时间轻度增加（不完全 RBBB），V5 ~V6 有较深的 S 波。

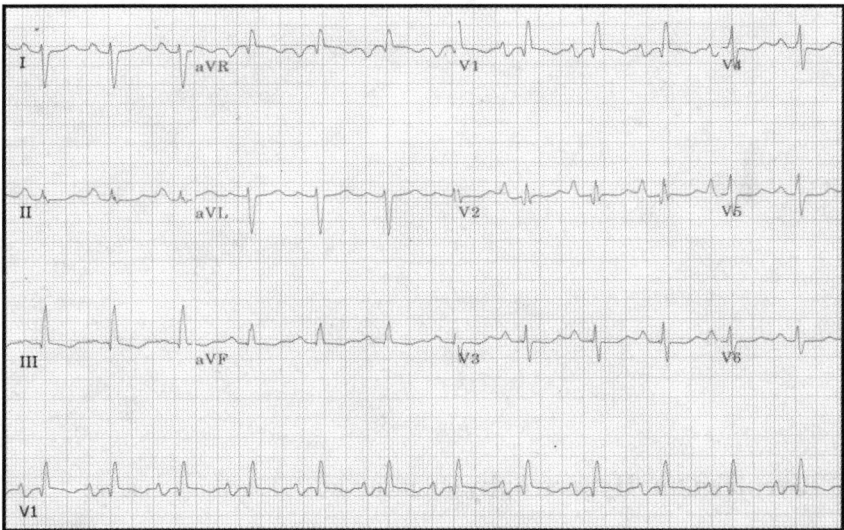

图 8 – 3

例2：18 岁患有原发性肺动脉高压的患者。注意：明显的电轴右偏（ +140°），R V1 >7mm，V1 ~ V3 导联明显向前的向量，RAE 的 P 波振幅增加，而且胸前导联典型的右心室压力型（ST 压低，T 波倒置）。

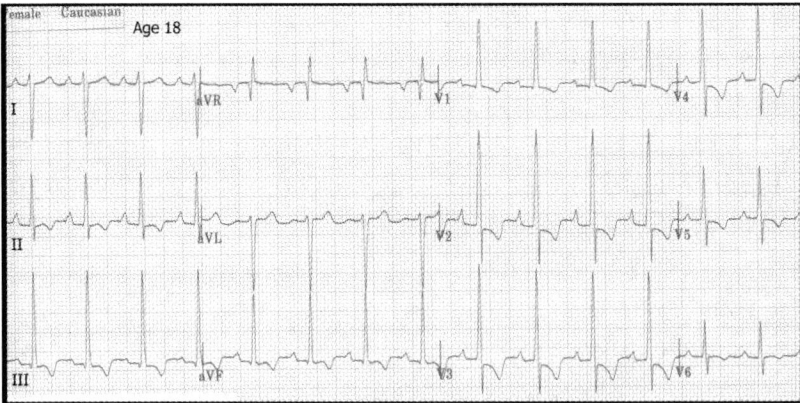

Fig. 8 – 4

Example 3: RVH in patient with an atrial septal defect. Note the incomplete RBBB pattern in V1 (rsR′), and the slight RAD (+105°).

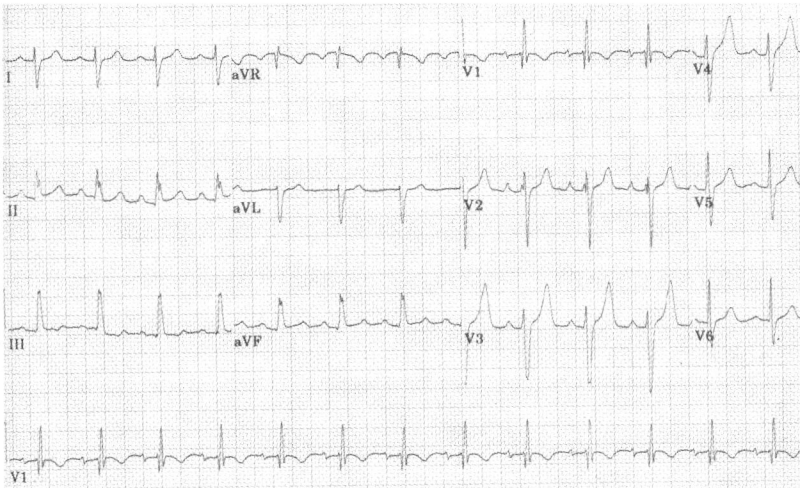

Fig. 8 – 5

8.3 Biventricular Hypertrophy (difficult ECG diagnosis to make)

(1) In the presence of LAE any one of the following suggests this diagnosis:

- R/S ratio in V5 or V6 < 1
- S in V5 or V6 > 6 mm
- RAD (> 90°)

(2) Other suggestive ECG findings:

- Criteria for LVH and RVH both metor LVH criteria met and RAD or RAE

present

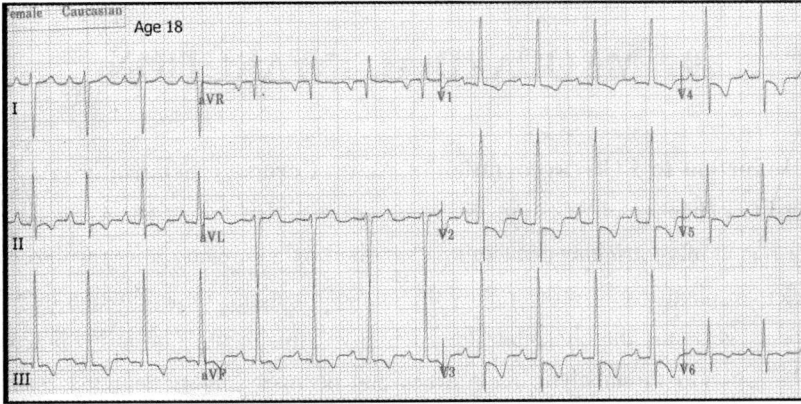

图 8－4

例 3：房间隔缺损伴右心室大的患者。注意 V1 是不完全 RBBB（rsR′），而且轻度电轴右偏（+105°）。

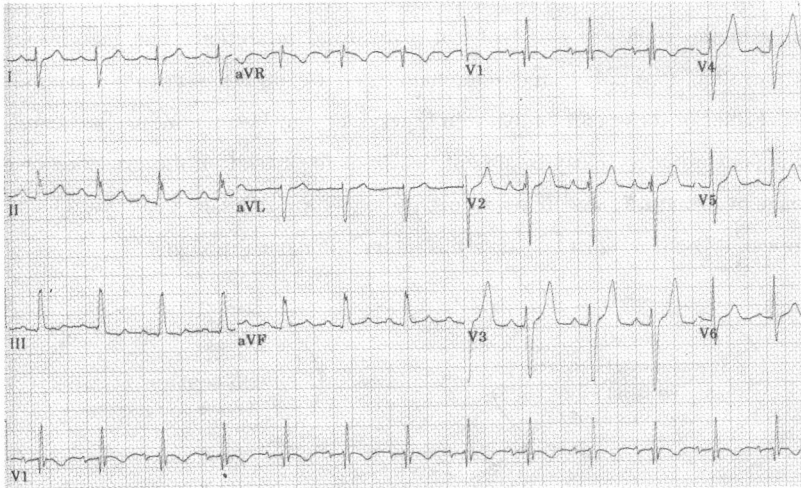

图 8－5

8.3　双心室肥大（凭心电图诊断有难度）

（1）左心房大 + 下列任何 1 条提示可以诊断：

- R/S V5 或 V6 <1。
- S V5 或 V6 >6 mm。
- 电轴右偏（>90°）。

（2）其他提示双心室肥大的心电图表现有：

- LVH 和 RVH 的标准都符合或符合 LVH 标准伴电轴右偏或存在 RAE。

9 MYOCARDIAL INFARCTION

Introduction to ECG Recognition of Acute Coronary Syndrome（ACS）

The ECG changes of ACS are the result of a sudden reduction of coronary blood flow to a region of ventricular myocardium supplied by a coronary artery with a ruptured atherosclerotic plaque and intracoronary thrombus formation. Depending on how quickly the patient gets to the hospital for definitive treatment（usually percutaneous revascularization or thrombolytic Rx）myocardial necrosis（infarction）may or may not occur. The diagram in Fig. 9 – 1 shows four possible ECG outcomes of myocardial ischemia in the setting of an acute coronary syndrome. On the left side no myocardial necrosis occurs but there is eithersubendocardial ischemia manifested by reversible ST segment depression or transmural ischemia manifested by reversible ST segment elevation. On the right are two types of myocardial infarction, one manifested by ST segment elevation（STEMI）and one manifested by no ST segment elevation（Non-STEMI）. Either of these can evolve into Q-wave or non-Q-wave MI's. Because Q waves may not appear initially, early treatment decisions are based on the presence or absence of ST segment elevation, and if revascularization is accomplished quickly Q-waves may never appear（"time is muscle" says the interventional cardiologist）.

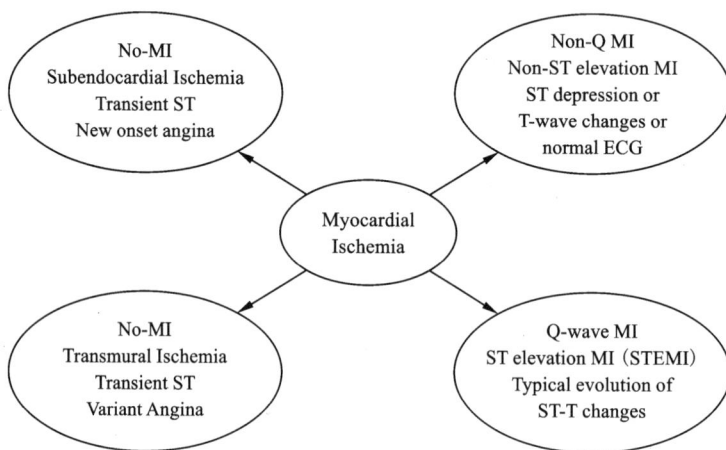

Fig. 9 – 1

9 心肌梗死

心电图如何识别急性冠状动脉综合征（ACS）

ACS 的心电图变化是由于冠状动脉粥样硬化斑块破裂和血栓形成导致冠状动脉对该区域的心肌组织供应的血流突然减少而形成的。这取决于快速的将患者送到医院并立即得到明确的治疗（通常是经皮血管再成形治疗或溶栓治疗），心肌坏死（梗死）可能会或可能不会发生。图 9 – 1 显示了急性冠脉综合征心肌缺血的四个可能的心电图结果。左边没有心肌坏死发生但表现为**心内膜**下心肌缺血见可逆的 ST 段压低，或**透壁**的缺血表现为可逆的 ST 段抬高。右边是两种类型的心肌梗死，一个体现为 ST 段抬高（STEMI），一个体现为无 ST 段抬高（Non-STEMI）。两者都可以演变成 Q 波型或非 Q 波型心肌梗死。因为 Q 波最初可能不会出现，早期治疗的决定是基于 ST 段抬高的存在与否，如果血管再成形快速完成 Q 波可能永远不会出现（介入心脏病学家铭言"**时间就是心肌**"）。

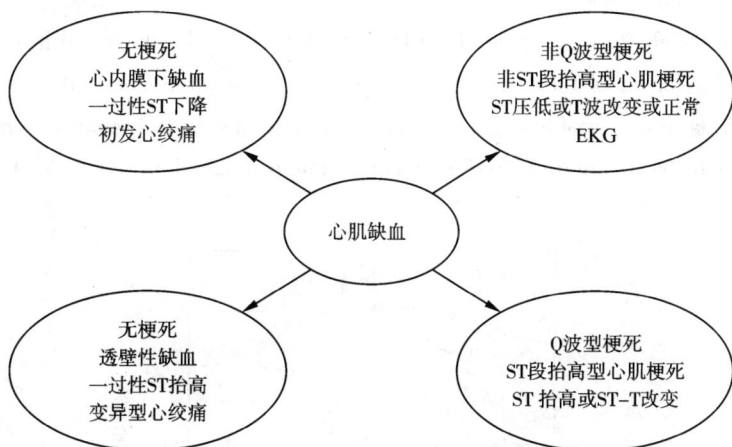

图 9 – 1

The following discussion will focus on ECG changes during the evolution of a STEMI.

- All MI's involve thel eft ventricular myocardium. In the setting of a proximal right coronary artery occlusion, however, there may also be a component of right ventricular infarction as well. Right sided chest leads are usually needed to recognize RV MI.

- In general, the more leads of the 12-lead ECG with MI changes (Q waves and/ or ST elevation), the larger the infarct size and the worse the prognosis (i. e. , more damage).

- The left anterior descending coronary artery (LAD) and it's branches supply the anterior and anterolateral walls of the left ventricle and the anterior two-thirds of the septum. The left circumflex coronary artery (LCx) and its branches supply the posterolateral wall of the left ventricle. The right coronary artery (RCA) supplies the right ventricle, as well as the inferior (diaphragmatic) and posterior-lateral walls of the left ventricle, and the posterior third of the septum. The RCA also gives off the AV nodal coronary artery in 85% – 90% of individuals; in the remaining 10% – 15% , this artery is a branch of the LCX.

- The usual ECG evolution of a STEMI with Q-waves is illustrated in the diagram in Fig. 9 – 2. Not all of the 6 patterns may be seen; the time from onset of MI to the final pattern is quite variable and is related to the size of MI, the rapidity of reperfusion (if any), and the location of the MI. (This example might be seen in lead Ⅱ during an acute inferior MI)

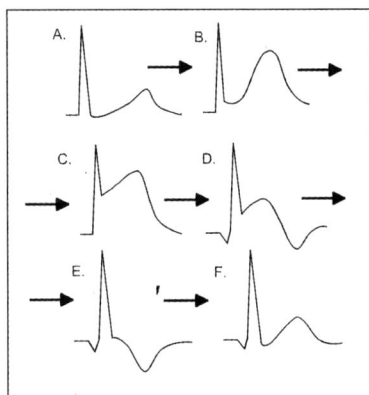

Evolution of Acute MI

Fig. 9 – 2

下列讨论集中在 ST 段抬高型心肌梗死（STEMI）演变的心电图变化。

● 所有的心肌梗死都会累及到**左心室心肌**，但是右冠状动脉近端堵塞时 **右心室梗死**是主要成分，常常需要用右胸导联去识别右心室心肌梗死。

● 一般来说，在 12 导联中涉及到心肌梗死变化（Q 波和/或 ST 抬高）的导联 越多，梗死面积越大，预后越差（即心肌损伤越多）。左前降支冠状动脉（LAD）及 其分支供应左心室前壁和前侧壁以及室间隔前 2/3 的血液；左回旋支冠状动脉 （LCX）及其分支供应左心室后侧壁的血液；右冠状动脉（RCA）供应右心室血液， 也供应下壁（膈面）和后侧壁以及室间隔后 1/3 的血液。人群中 85% ~ 90% 的房 室结由 RCA 供血；剩余的 10% ~ 15% 由 LCX 的分支供血。

● 伴有 Q 波的 STEMI 的心电图一般演变过程如图 9 - 2 所示。不是所有的 6 种模式都可以见到；从心肌梗死发作到最终模式形成的时间变化非常大，取决于 梗死（MI）的大小，再灌注（如果有的话）的速度和梗死的位置（如急性下壁心肌梗 死心电图的 Ⅱ 导联所见）。

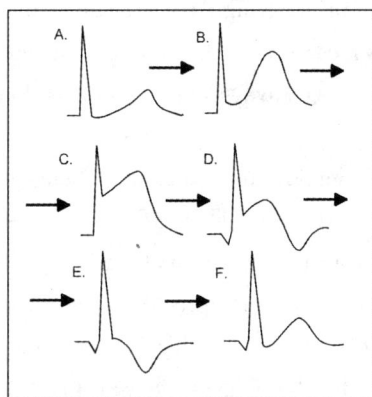

急性心肌梗死的心电图演变

图 9 - 2

A. Normal ECG prior to the onset of plaque rupture

B. Hyperacute T wave changes-increased T wave amplitude and width; QT prolongs; may also see some ST segment elevation

C. Marked ST elevation with hyperacute T wave changes ("tombstone" pattern)

D. Pathologic Q waves appear (necrosis), ST elevation decreases, T waves begin to invert (this is also called the "fully evolved" phase)

E. Pathologic Q waves, T wave inversion (necrosis and fibrosis)

F. Pathologic Q waves, upright T waves (fibrosis)

(G). Q waves may get smaller or disappear with time

9.1 Inferior MI Family of STEMI's (Q-wave MI's)

includes inferior, true posterior, and right ventricular MI's.

- Inferior MI

- Pathologic Q waves and evolving ST – T changes in leads Ⅱ, Ⅲ, aVF

- Q waves (if they appear) are usually largest in lead Ⅲ, next largest in lead aVF, and smallest in lead Ⅱ. Q wave ≥30ms in aVF is diagnostic.

Example 1: Acute inferior MI injury pattern. Note hyperacute T waves with ST elevation in Ⅱ, Ⅲ, aVF (ST↑ in Ⅲ > ST↑ in Ⅱ suggests RCA occlusion); reciprocal ST depression is seen in Ⅰ, and aVL. ST depression in V1 – V3 represents true posterior injury pattern and not a reciprocal change (see true posterior MI patterns below). The V4 and V5 electrode sites in this ECG are interchanged (this is an ECG technician error; it doesn't alter the diagnosis however).

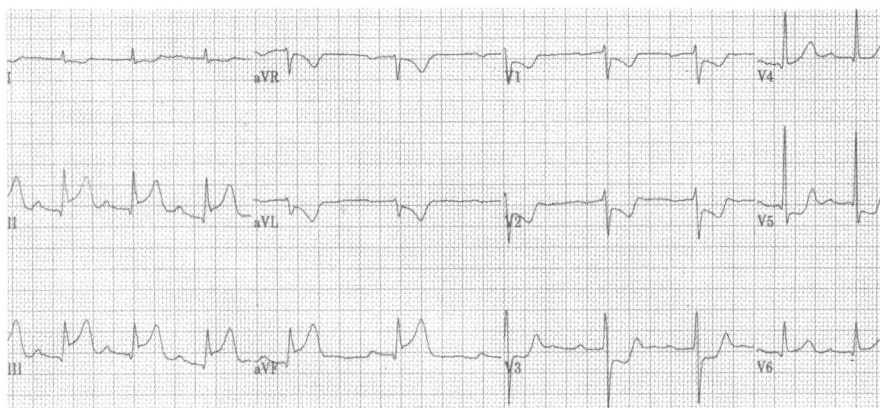

Fig. 9 – 3

A. 出现斑块破裂之前的正常心电图。

B. 超急性期 T 波变化——T 波幅度和宽度增加;QT 延长,也可以看到一些 ST 段抬高。

C. 明显的 ST 段抬高伴超急性期 T 波变化("墓碑"型)。

D. 病理性 Q 波出现(坏死)、ST 段回落下降,T 波开始倒置(这也被称为"充分演变"阶段)。

E. 病理性 Q 波,T 波倒置(坏死和纤维化)。

F. 病理性 Q 波,T 波直立(纤维化)。

(G)Q 波可能随着时间变小或消失。

9.1 STEMI's 的下壁心肌梗死家族(Q 波型心肌梗死)

包括下壁,正后壁和右心室心肌梗死。

- 下壁梗死。
- Ⅱ,Ⅲ,aVF 病理性 Q 波和 ST – T 变化的演变。
- Q 波(如果他们出现)通常是最大的在 Ⅲ 导联,其次在 aVF,最小的在 Ⅱ 导联,aVF 的 Q 波≥30 ms 诊断成立。

例1:急性下壁心肌梗死损伤模式。注意 Ⅱ,Ⅲ,aVF 导联的超急性期 T 波和抬高的 ST 段(ST↑ Ⅲ > ST↑ Ⅱ 表明 RCA 闭塞);Ⅰ 和 aVL 的 ST 段反而压低(镜像改变)。V1 ~ V3 导联 ST 段压低代表正后壁损伤模式,而不是镜像改变(参见下面的正后壁 MI 模式)。V4 和 V5 在这个心电图电极位置应该互换(这是一个心电图技术错误;但是它不改变诊断)。

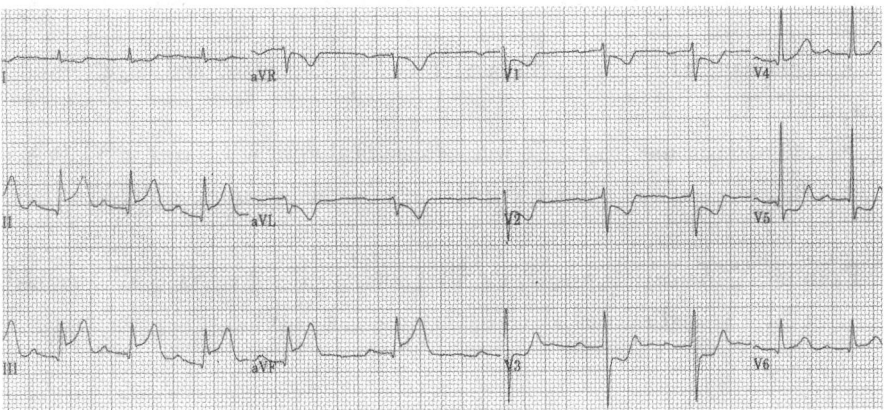

图 9 – 3

Example 2：Old inferior MI（note largest Q in lead Ⅲ, next largest in aVF, and smallest in lead Ⅱ）. Axis = −50°（LAD）; T wave inversion is also present in leads Ⅱ, Ⅲ, and aVF.

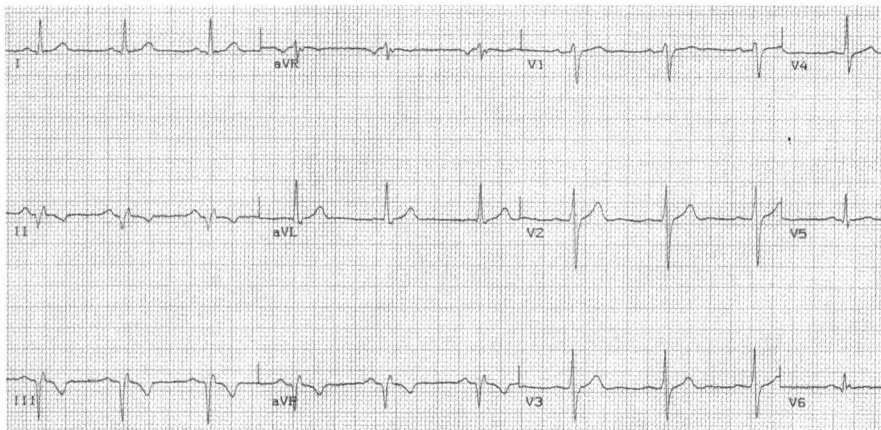

Fig. 9 −4

True posterior MI：ECG changes are seen in precordial leads V1 − V3, but are the mirror image of an anteroseptal MI（because the posterior wall is behind the anterior wall）

● Increased R wave amplitude and/or duration ≥40 ms in V1 − V2（i. e., a "pathologic R wave" is the mirror image of a pathologic Q on the posterior wall-seen in V8 and V9）

● R/S ratio in V1 or V2 >1（i. e., prominent anterior forces; need to R/O RVH）

● Hyperacute ST − T wave changes：i. e., ST depression and large, inverted T waves in V1`− V3

● Late normalization of ST − T with symmetrical upright T waves in V1 to V3

● Often seen with an inferior wall MI（i. e., "infero-posterior MI"）

Example 3：Acute infero-posterior MI（note tall R waves V1 − V3, marked ST depression V1 −3, and inferior ST elevation in Ⅱ, Ⅲ, aVF）

例2：陈旧下壁心肌梗死（注意Ⅲ导联Q波最大，其次在 aVF，Ⅱ导联最小）。电轴 = −50°（左偏）；Ⅱ，Ⅲ和 aVF 导联也存在着 T 波倒置。

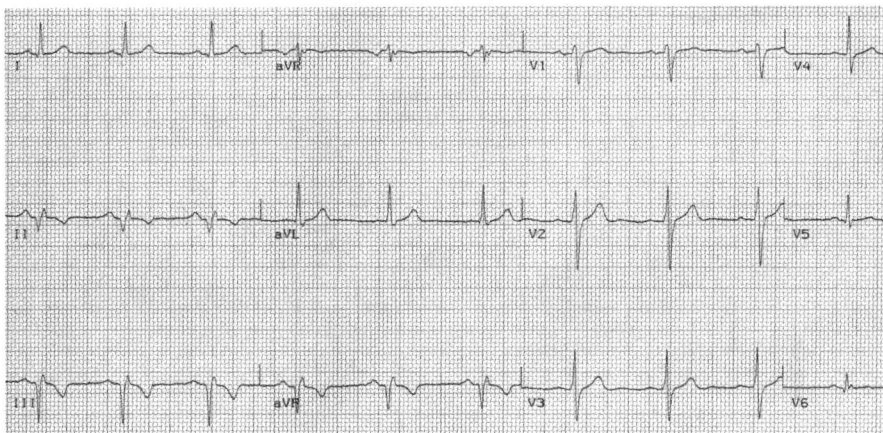

图 9 − 4

正后壁梗死：心电图改变见胸前 V1 ~ V3 导联，但是与前间隔梗死呈镜像表现（因为后壁在前壁之后）

- V1 ~ V2 导联 R 波振幅增加和/或时间 ≥40 ms（即与 V8 和 V9 导联病理性 Q 波形成镜像的一个"病理性 R 波"）。
- R/S V1 或 V2 >1（即明显向前的向量；需要除外 RVH）。
- 超急性期 ST − T 的变化：即 ST 段压低和 V1 ~ V3 导联大的倒置的 T 波。
- V1 到 V3 导联 ST − T 后来正常化伴有直立的对称 T 波。
- 通常见到下壁心肌梗死（即"下后壁心肌梗死"）。

例3：急性下后壁心肌梗死（注意 V1 − 3 所有的高的 R 波伴明显的 ST 段压低，而且下壁的Ⅱ，Ⅲ，aVF 导联 ST 段抬高）

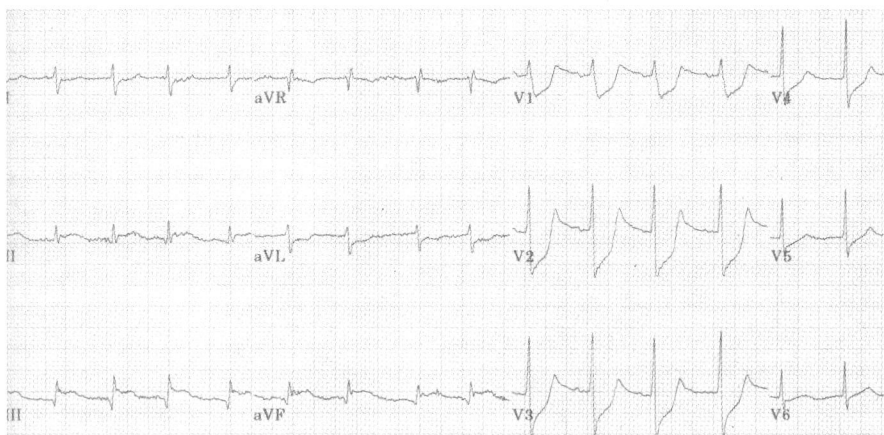

Fig. 9 – 5

Example 4：Old infero-posterior MI：Note tall，wide pathologic R in V1 – V3（this is a Q wave equivalent），upright T waves，and inferior Q waves with residual ST segment elevation）

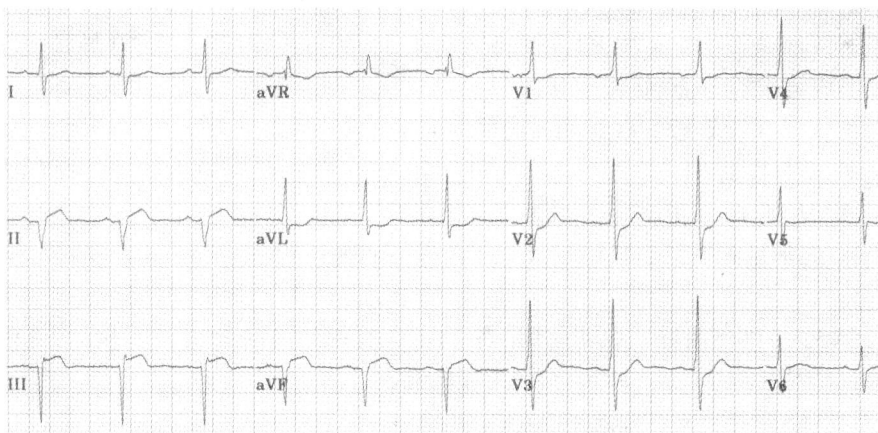

Fig. 9 – 6

Differential Diagnosis of Tall R waves in V1 or V2（and narrow QRS complexes）：

- True posterior myocardial infarction（see above）
- Right ventricular hypertrophy（p133）
- Left septal fascicular block（a controversial diagnosis）
- Normal variant
- Misplaced precordial leads

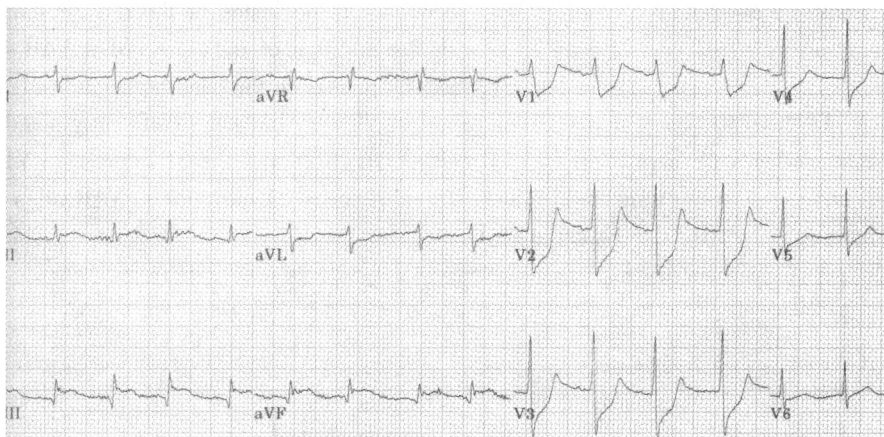

图 9-5

例 4：陈旧下后壁心肌梗死[注意 V1-3 导联所有的高的、宽的病理性 R 波（这等同于病理性 Q 波），直立的 T 波和下壁的 Q 波伴残留的 ST 段抬高]

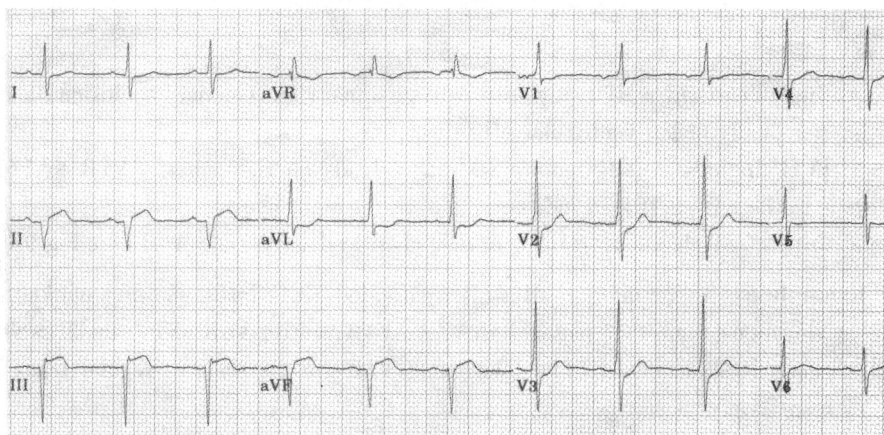

图 9-6

V1 或 V2 高 R 波的鉴别诊断（和窄的 QRS 波群）：

- 正后壁心肌梗死（见上文内容）
- 右心室肥大（p134）
- 左前分支阻滞（有争议的诊断）
- 正常变异
- 胸前导联错位

Example 5: Acute "posterior MI" secondary to occlusion of the left circumflex coronary artery. This is a 15-lead ECG with the addition of right precordial V4R (to diagnose RV MI), and posterior leads V8 and V9 placed on the back horizontal to leads V4 – 6. In this ECG one can see ST elevation in V8 – 9, but not significantly noted in the standard leads (except, perhaps, Ⅰ and aVL). Note also the ST depression V1 – 6 indicative of posterior transmural injury. The absence of ST elevation in V4R rules out a right ventricular MI (see Example #6 below).

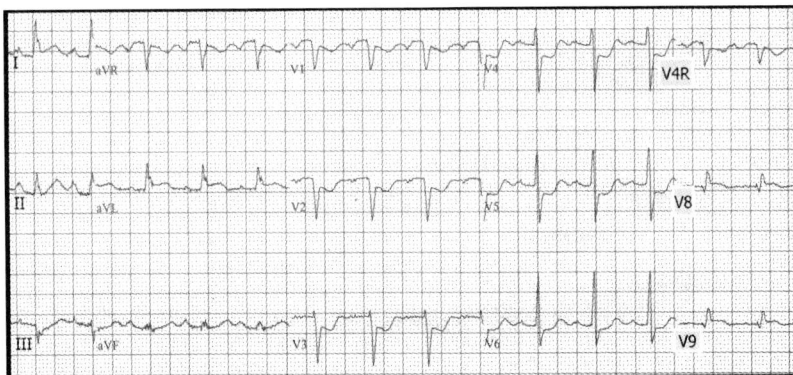

Fig. 9 – 7

● Right Ventricular MI (only seen with proximal right coronary occlusion; i. e. , with inferior family of left ventricular MI's)

· ECG findings usually require additional leads on right chest (V1R to V6R, analogous to the left chest lead locations, but on the right chest)

· Criteria: ST elevation, ≥1mm, in right chest leads, especially V4R (see Fig. 9 – 8)

Example 6: Acute inferior MI with right-sided ECG leads showing marked ST segment elevation (tombstone pattern) in V3R, V4R, V5R, V6R. ST↑ in Ⅲ > ST↑ in Ⅱ suggests RCA occlusion. (note V1R and V2R are the same as regular leads V2 and V1 respectively)

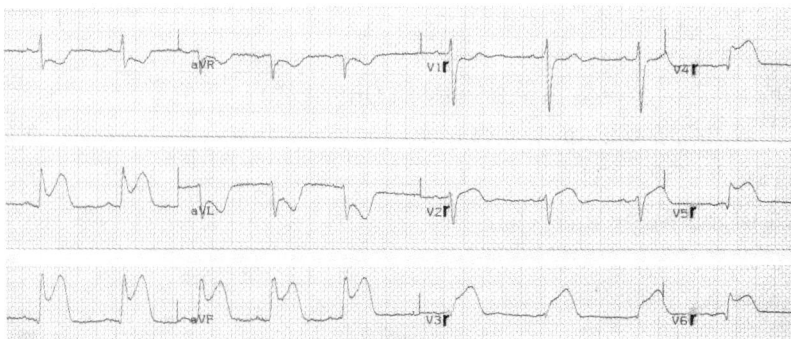

Fig. 9 – 8

例5：急性"后壁心肌梗死"继发于冠状动脉左回旋支闭塞。图 9 - 7 是一个 15 导联心电图，增加了右心前导联 V4R（诊断右心室心肌梗死），和后面 V8 和 V9 导联放置在 V4 ~ V6 水平。在这个心电图可以看到后壁导联 V8 ~ V9 的 ST 段抬高，但标准导联没有明显的看到（除外 Ⅰ 和 aVL）。还要注意 V1 ~ V6 的 ST 段压低表明后壁透壁性损伤。V4R 的 ST 段没有抬高排除了右心室心肌梗死（参见下面的例6）。

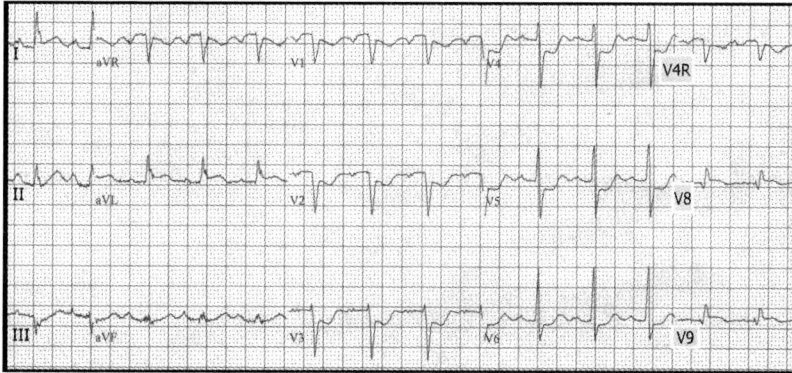

图 9 - 7

● 右心室心肌梗死（仅见于近端右冠状动脉闭塞；也就是说，伴有左心室下壁的心肌梗死）

· 心电图观察通常需要额外的右胸导联（V1R ~ V6R，类似于左胸导联位置，但在右边的胸部）。

· 标准：ST 段抬高≥1mm，在右胸导联，特别是 V4R（见图 9 - 8）。

例6：急性下壁心肌梗死，伴有右侧胸前导联 V3R，V4R，V5R，V6R 的 ST 段明显抬高（墓碑模式）。ST↑ Ⅲ ＞ST↑ Ⅱ 表明 RCA 阻塞。（注意 V1R 和 V2R 分别同常规 V2 和 V1 导联相对应。）

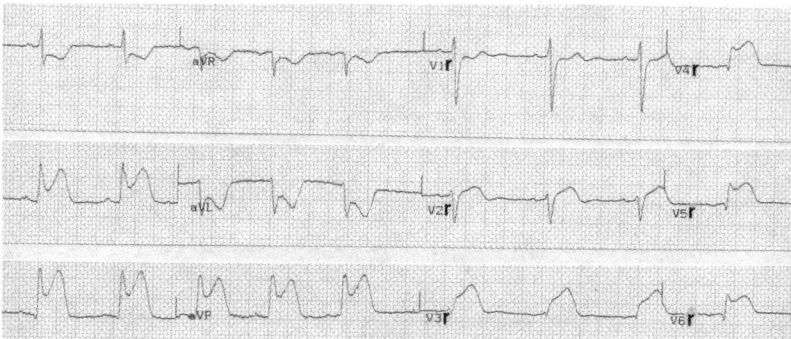

图 9 - 8

9.2 Anterior Family of STEMI's

includes anteroseptal, anterior, anterolateral, and high lateral
- Anteroseptal MI
  - Q, QS, or qrS complexes in leads V1 – V3 (V4)
  - Evolving ST – T changes

Example #7: Hyperacute anteroseptal MI; marked ST elevation in V1 – V3 before Q waves developed (note convex-up ST elevation in V1 – 3)

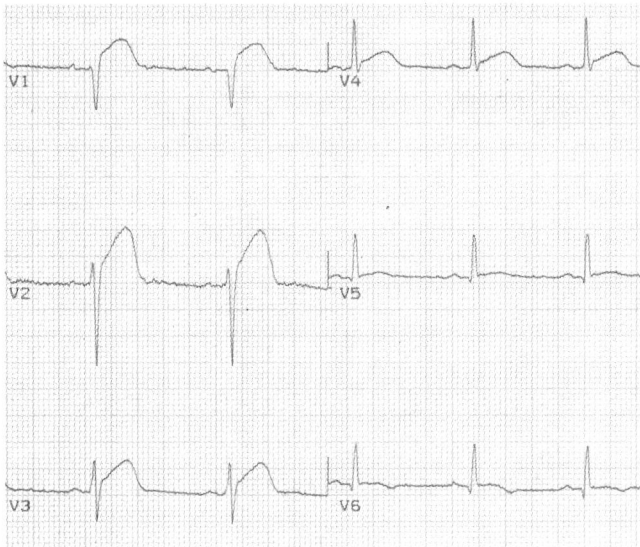

Fig. 9 – 9

Example #8: Fully evolved anteroseptal MI (note QS waves in V1 – V2, qrS complex in V3, plus ST – T wave changes)

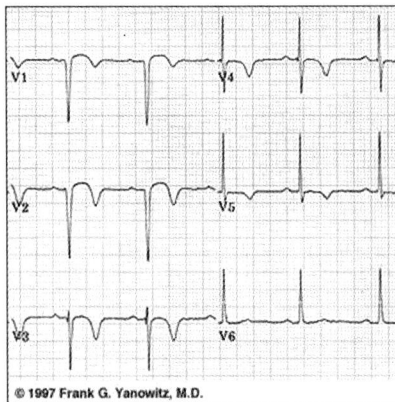

© 1997 Frank G. Yanowitz, M.D.

Fig. 9 – 10

9.2　STEMI's 的前壁梗死家族

　　STEMI's 的前壁梗死家族包括前间隔，前壁，前侧壁和高侧壁。
- 前间壁心肌梗死
- ·V1 ~ V3(V4)导联呈 Q，QS 或 qrS 波形。
- ·ST – T 改变的演变

　　例7：超急性期的前间壁心肌梗死；V1 ~ V3 的 ST 段在 Q 波形成之前明显抬高(注意 V1 ~ V3 的 ST 段呈弓背向上抬高)。

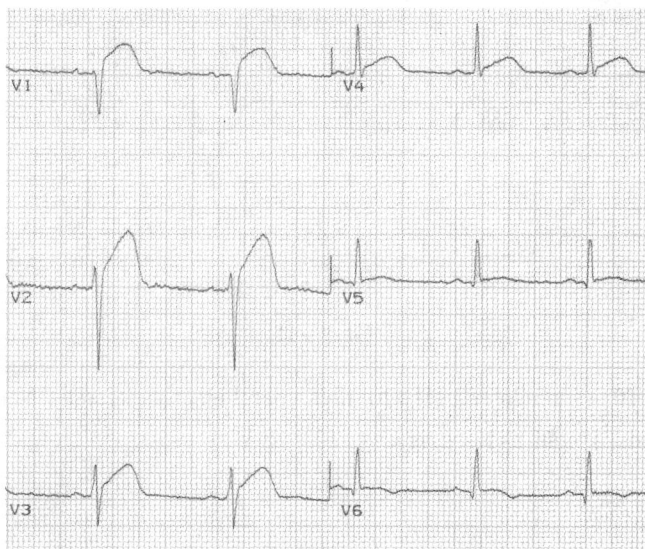

图9 – 9

　　例8：前间隔心肌梗死的充分演变(注意 V1 ~ V2 的 QS 波，V3 的 qrS，加 ST – T 改变)

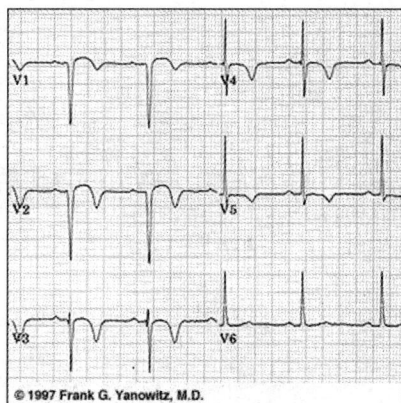

© 1997 Frank G. Yanowitz, M.D.

图9 – 10

• Anterior MI (similar changes, but usually V1 is spared; if V4 – 6 involved call it "anterolateral"; if changes also in leads Ⅰ and aVL it's a "high-lateral" MI.

Example 9：Acute Anterolateral injury; note ST elevation V3 – 6. Possible inferior MI also present of uncertain age.

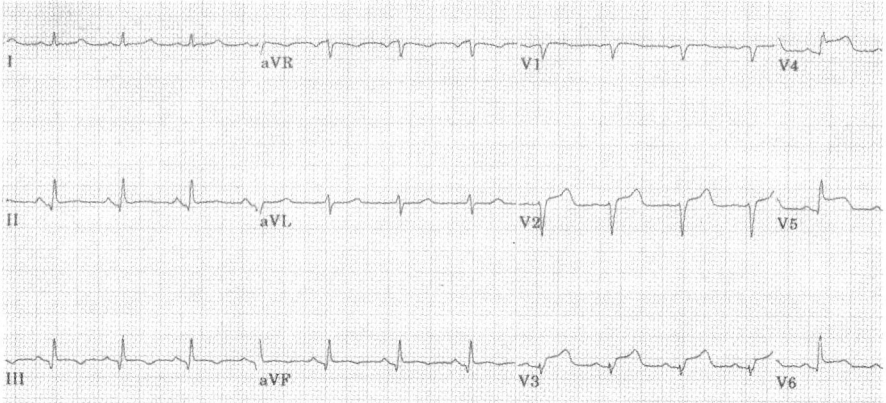

Fig. 9 – 11

Example 10：Anterolateral MI with high lateral changes as well. Note Q's V2 – V6 plus Q's in leads Ⅰ and aVL. Axis = +120° (RAD)

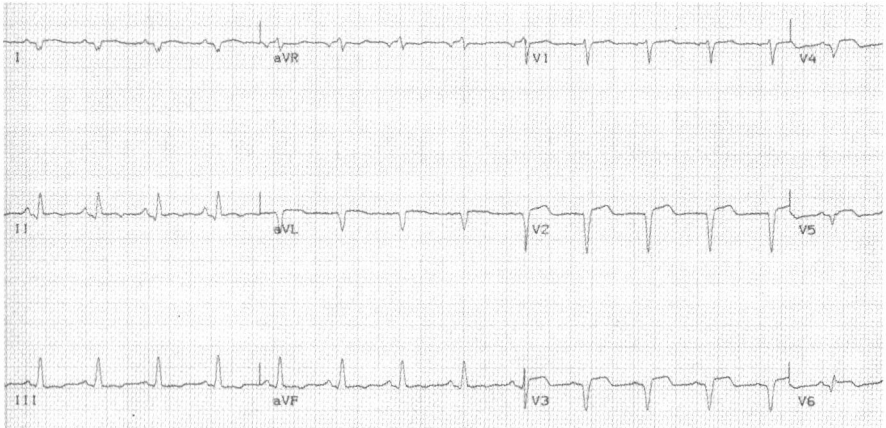

Fig. 9 – 12

● **前壁心肌梗死**：变化类似，但通常 V1 幸免，如果涉及到 V4 ～ V6 称之为"前侧壁"；如果变化也发生在 I 和 aVL 称"高侧壁"心肌梗死。

例9：急性**前侧壁**损伤；注意 V3 ～ V6 的 ST 段抬高。可能也存在不确定的时间的下壁心肌梗死。

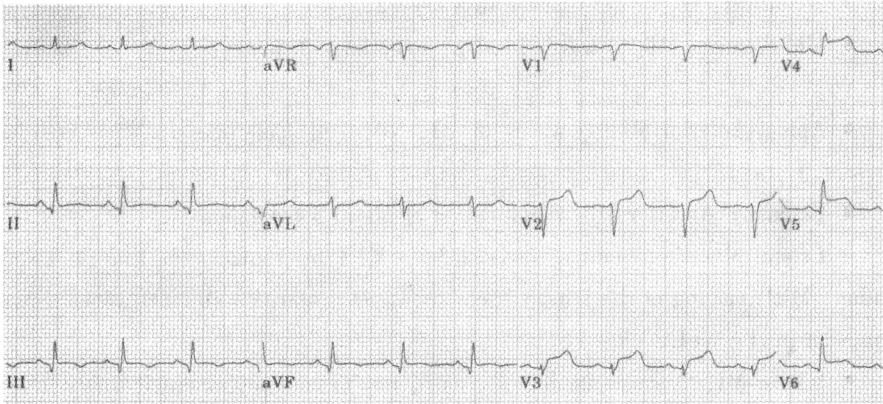

图 9 - 11

例10：前侧壁心肌梗死也伴有高侧壁的变化。注意 V2 ～ V6 的 Q's 加 I 和 aVL 的 Q's，电轴 = +120°（RAD）。

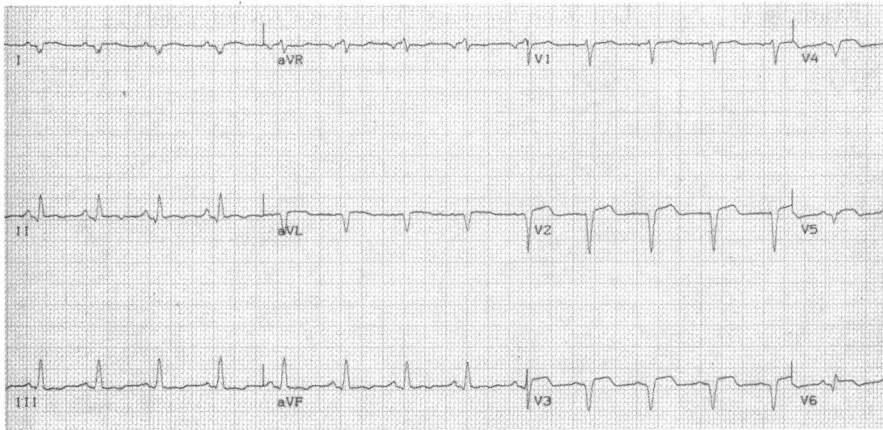

图 9 - 12

Comment：The precise identification of MI locations on the ECG is evolving as new heart imaging（e. g.，MRI）better defines the ventricular anatomy. New terminology has been suggested（see Circulation 2006；114：1755）. While not universally accepted, the following "new" Q-wave MI patterns have been defined for left ventricular segments seen on MRI imaging：

- Septal MI：Q（or QS）waves in V1 – V2
- Mid-Anterior MI：Q waves in aVL, sometimes in lead Ⅰ, V2, V3, but not in V5 – V6.
- Apical-Anterior MI：Q waves in V3, V4, and sometimes in V5 – V6. No Q waves in Ⅰ, aVL
- Extensive Anterior MI：Combination of above 3 locations.
- Lateral MI：Prominent R waves in V1 – V2（this replaces the true posterior MI location；MRI imaging of the left ventricle shows no posterior wall）. Q waves may also be present in Ⅰ, aVL, V5 – V6.
- Inferor MI：Q waves in Ⅱ, Ⅲ, aVF, but without prominent R waves in V1 – V2

（It remains to be seen whether or not this new terminology of infarct location will become accepted in the ECG literature of the future）

Example 11：Acute Left Main Coronary Occlusion（pay attention！）：

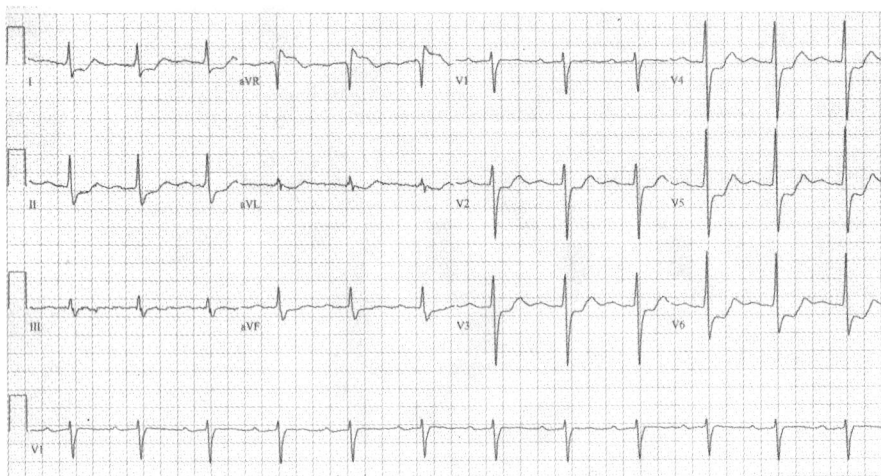

Fig. 9 – 13

● 备注：心电图对心肌梗死的精确定位正在演变为新的心脏成像（如磁共振成像 MRI），更好地定义了心室解剖，虽然目前还没有被普遍接受，新的术语已经被建议（见 2006 循环杂志；114：1755）。下面磁共振成像定义了左心室各部分的"新"Q 波心肌梗死模式：

● 间隔心肌梗死：V1 ~ V2 导联的 Q 波或 QS 波。

● 中前壁心肌梗死：aVL 为 Q 波，有时见于 I，V2，V3，但是 V5 ~ V6 没有。

● 心尖前壁心肌梗死：Q V3，Q V4，有时 Q V5 ~ V6，I、aVL 导联没有 Q 波。

● 广泛前壁心肌梗死：包括以上 3 个部位。

● 侧壁心肌梗死：V1 ~ V2 导联 R 波明显（这一点类似正后壁心肌梗死；但左心室的 MRI 成像证实没有正后壁），I，aVL，V5 ~ V6 也可以有 Q 波存在。

● 下壁心肌梗死：Q II，III，aVF，但是 V1 ~ V2 没有明显的 R 波。

（这些梗死部位新的术语是否会被将来的心电图文献所接受还有待于观察）

例 11：急性左主干闭塞（高度关注！）

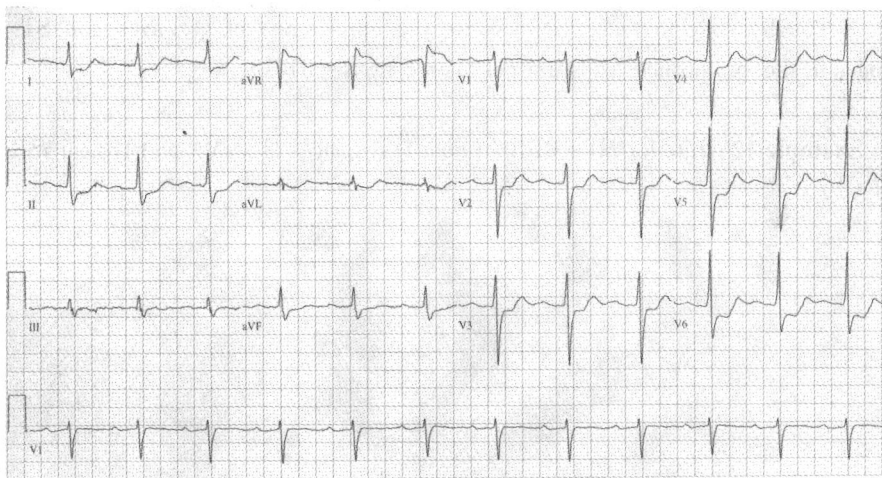

图 9 – 13

The ECG illustrated above is a tragic case of missed acute left main coronary occlusion. It was missed diagnosed as a non-STEMI because of the absence of typical ST segment elevation in 2 or more contiguous ECG leads. Instead of proceeding to emergent coronary intervention, the patient was treated with the non-STEMI protocol in the CCU for 12 hrs until a disastrous cardiac arrest occurred. The ECG findings of left main coronary occlusion seen in the above ECG include:

- ST segment elevation in aVR > any ST elevation in V1
- ST segment depression in 7 or more leads of the 12-lead ECG
- This ECG is considered a STEMI equivalent and should be Rx'ed emergently.

Similar ECG findings may occur in acute MI due to severe 3-vessel coronary artery disease.

9.3 MI with Bundle Branch Block

9.3.1 MI + Right Bundle Branch Block

· Usually easy to recognize because the appearance of Q waves and ST – T changes in the appropriate leads are not altered by the RBBB

Example 12: Inferior MI + RBBB (note Q's in Ⅱ, Ⅲ, aVF and typical rSR′ in lead V1)

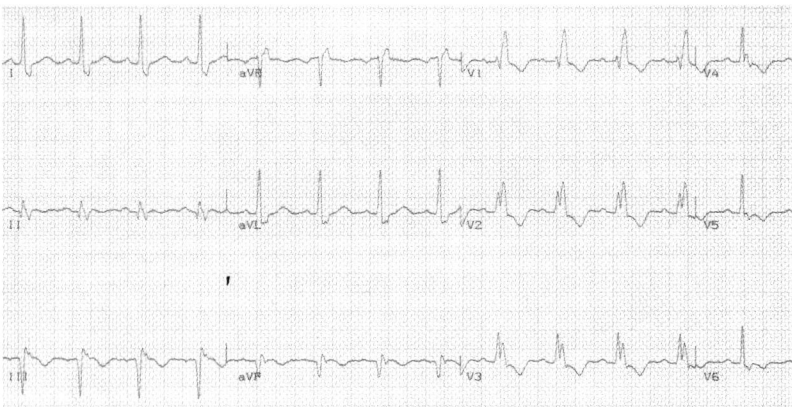

Fig. 9 – 14

Example 13: Extensive anterior MI with RBBB + LAFB; note pathologic Q's in leads V1 – V5, terminal fat R wave in V1 – V4, fat S wave in V6 of RBBB. Axis = – 80° (rS in Ⅱ, Ⅲ, and aVF: indicative of left anterior fascicular block; RBBB + LAFB indicates bifascicular block).

图9-13的心电图所示，是一个没有及时确认的悲剧性的急性左主冠状动脉阻塞。由于2个或更多连续的心电图导联缺乏典型的ST段抬高导致错误诊断为non-STEMI，因此没有进行紧急冠状动脉介入治疗，而是在冠心病监护病房（CCU）按照non-STEMI的处理程序治疗12小时直到一个灾难性的心脏骤停发生。

图9-13的心电图提示左主冠状动脉闭塞的特点包括：

- aVR的ST段抬高 > V1的任何一个抬高的ST段。
- 12导联心电图中ST段压低的导联≥7个。
- 这个心电图等同于STEMI，应该紧急救治。

类似心电图表现也可见于严重的3支冠状动脉病变的急性心肌梗死。

9.3 心肌梗死合并束支阻滞

9.3.1 心肌梗死+右束支传导阻滞（RBBB）

心肌梗死合并右束支传导阻滞通常容易辨认，因为相应的导联存在Q波和ST-T改变，这些并没有因为RBBB而改变。

例12：下壁心肌梗死+RBBB（注意Q's Ⅱ，Ⅲ，aVF和典型的rSR′ V1）

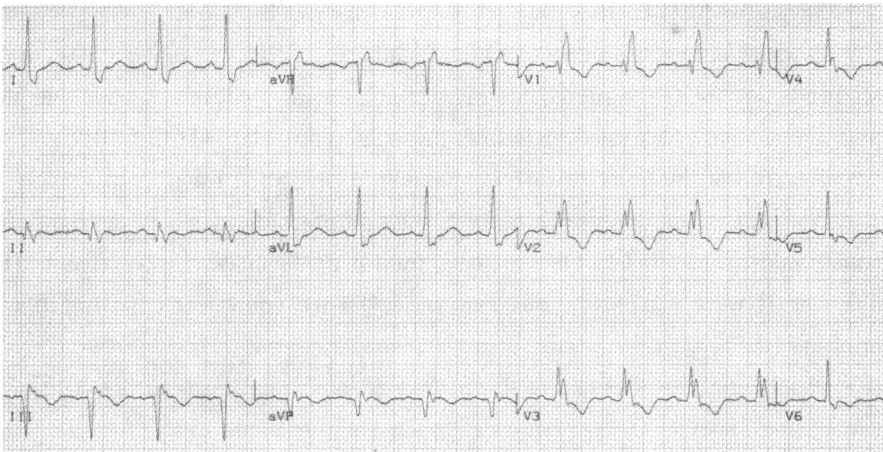

图9-14

例13：广泛前壁心肌梗死合并RBBB+LAFB。注意V1～V5病理性Q波，V1～V4终末胖R，V6胖S波。电轴 = -80°[Ⅱ，Ⅲ，aVF的rS的rS：左前分支阻滞（LAFB）；RBBB+LAFB是双分支阻滞]。

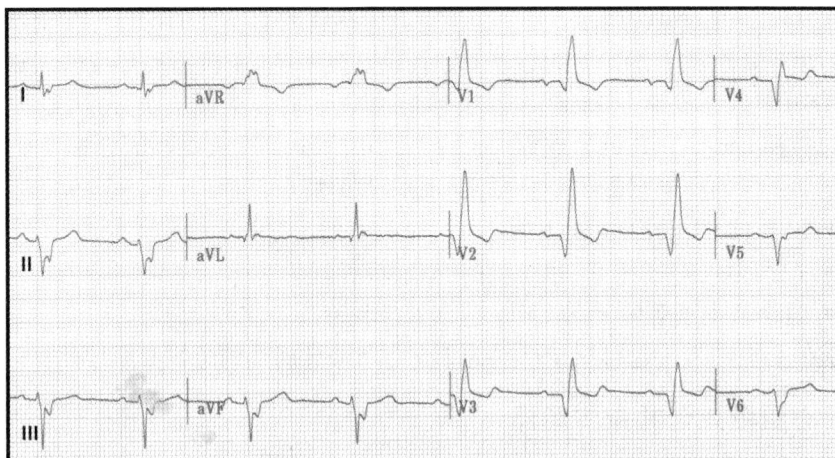

Fig. 9 – 15

9.3.2 MI + Left Bundle Branch Block

• Often a difficult ECG diagnosis because in LBBB the right ventricle is activated first and left ventricular infarct Q waves may not appear at the beginning of the QRS complex (unless the septum is involved).

• Suggested ECG features, not all of which are specific for MI include:

· Q waves of any size intwo or more of leads Ⅰ, aVL, V5, or V6 (See example 15 on P164: one of the most reliable signs and probably indicates septal infarction, because the septum is activated early from the right ventricular side in LBBB).

· Reversal of the usual R wave progression in precordial leads

· Notching of the downstroke of the S wave in precordial leads to the right of the transition zone (i. e., before QRS changes from a predominate S wave complex to a predominate R wave complex); this may be a Q-wave equivalent appearingafter the onset of the QRS.

· Notching of the upstroke of the S wave in precordial leads to the right of the transition zone (another Q-wave equivalent; see V4 in example 15).

· rSR′ complex in leads Ⅰ, V5 or V6 (the S is a Q-wave equivalent occurring in the middle of the QRS complex)

· RS complex in V5 – 6 rather than the usual monophasic R waves seen in uncomplicated LBBB; (the S is a Q-wave equivalent).

· "Primary" ST – T wave changes (i. e., ST – T changes in the same direction as the QRS complex rather than the usual "secondary" ST – T changes seen in uncomplicated LBBB); these changes may reflect an acute, evolving MI.

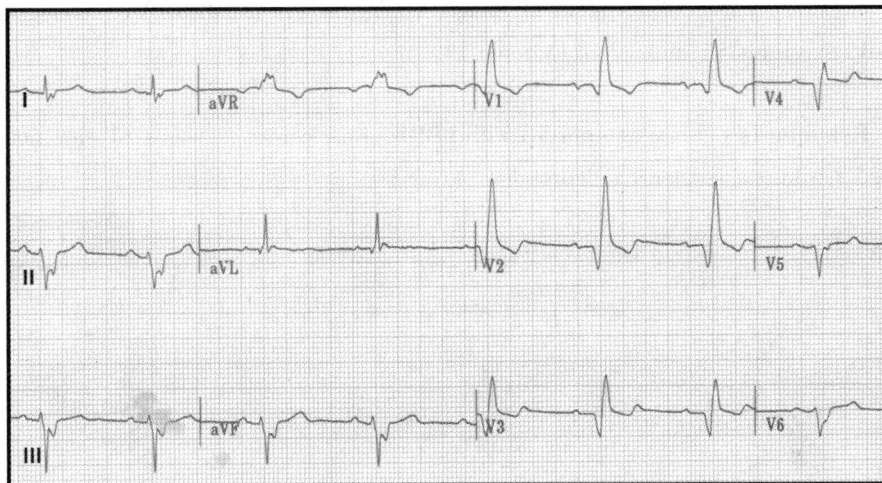

图 9 – 15

9.3.2 MI + 左束支传导阻滞(LBBB)

- 心电图诊断的困难常常因为在 LBBB 时右心室首先被激活,左心室梗死 Q 波可能不会出现在 QRS 波群的起始部(除非室间隔受累)。

- 以下为建议的心电图特征,并非所有的特征对心肌梗死都有特异性,包括:

· 在 Ⅰ,aVL,V5 或 V6 中有 2 个或以上导联有任何大小的 Q 波(参见心电图例 15,P165:这是最可靠的迹象之一,可能表明室间隔梗死,因为存在 LBBB 时从右心室侧首先兴奋室间隔)。

·· 胸前导联普通 R 波可逆性进展

· 胸前导联 S 波降支切迹向右区过渡(例如,QRS 变化之前从 S 波占主导变成以 R 波为主的综合波);这可能相当于是一个 QRS 出现后的 Q 波。

· 胸前导联 S 波升支切迹向右区过渡(另一个等效 Q 波;看例 15 的 V4 导联)。

· Ⅰ,V5 或 V6 为 rSR′(在 QRS 波群中间的 S 波相当于是 1 个 Q 波)

· 在 V5 ~ V6 导联是 RS 波群而不是通常在简单的 LBBB 所显示的单相 R 波(这个 S 波相当于 Q 波)。

· "原发性"ST – T 变化(例如,ST – T 改变与 QRS 波群在相同的方向,而不是那种简单常见的 LBBB 继发性 ST – T 改变),这些变化可能反映了一种急性、正在演变的心肌梗死。

· Exaggerated ST deviation in same direction as the usualLBBB ST changes in LBBB (see leads V1 and V2 in example 14).

Example 14: Acute anterior MI with LBBB. Note convex-upwards ST elevation in V1 – V3 with exaggerated ST depression in V – V6.

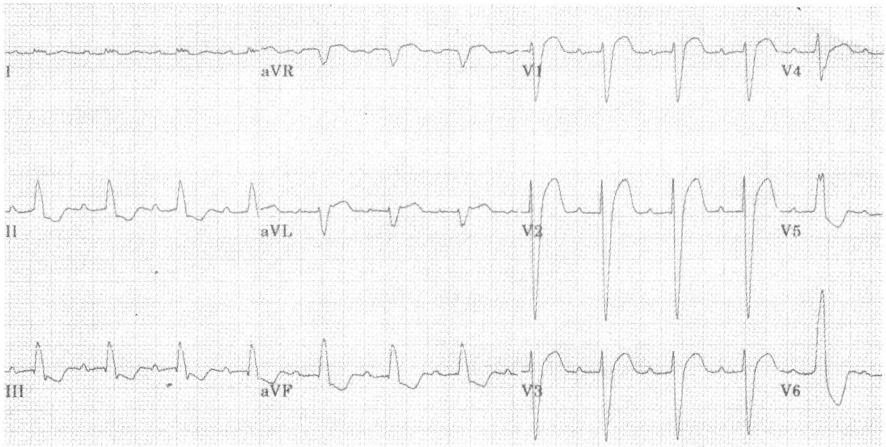

Fig. 9 – 16

Example 15: Old MI (probable septal location) with LBBB. Remember LBBB without MI should have monophasic R waves in Ⅰ, aVL, V6). This ECG has abnormal q waves in Ⅰ, aVL, V5 – V6 suggesting a septal MI location. Note also the notching on the upslope of S wave (arrow) in V4 ("sign of Cabrera") and the PVC couplet.

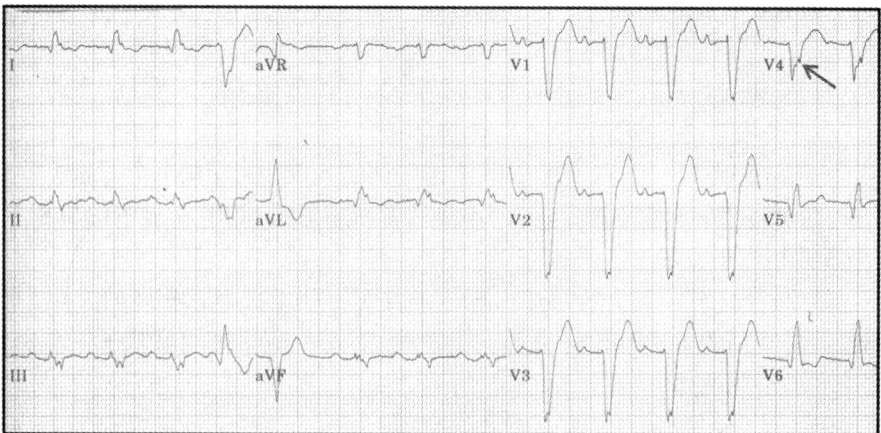

Fig. 9 – 17

· ST 改变与通常完全性左束支传导阻滞的 ST 改变方向相同，但很夸张（见例 14 的 V1 和 V2）。

例 14：急性前壁心肌梗死合并 LBBB。注意 V1 ~ V3 导联 ST 段弓背向上抬高，V6 导联 ST 段夸张性压低。

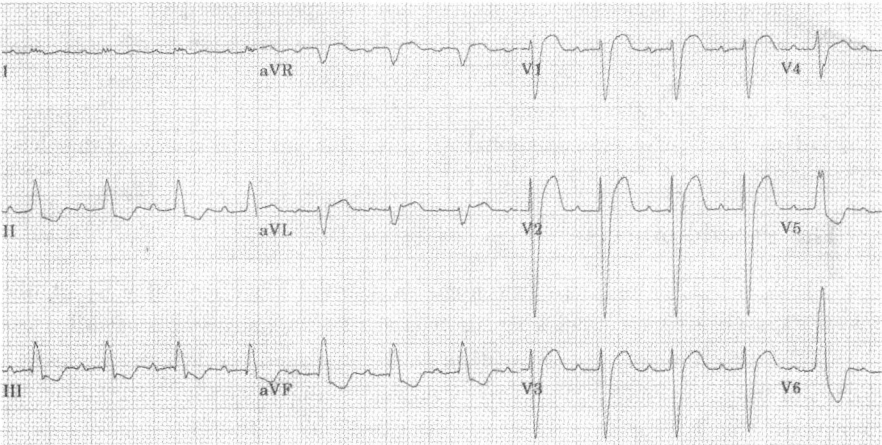

图 9 - 16

例 15：陈旧性心肌梗死（可能是室间隔）合并 LBBB。记住 LBBB 没有心肌梗死时在Ⅰ、aVL、V6 应该为单相 R 波。这个心电图Ⅰ、aVL、V5 ~ V6 导联有异常 Q 波提示心肌梗死位置在室间隔。还要注意 V4 导联 S 波斜形升支的切迹（箭头所示，"卡布瑞拉的迹象"）和成对的室性期前收缩。

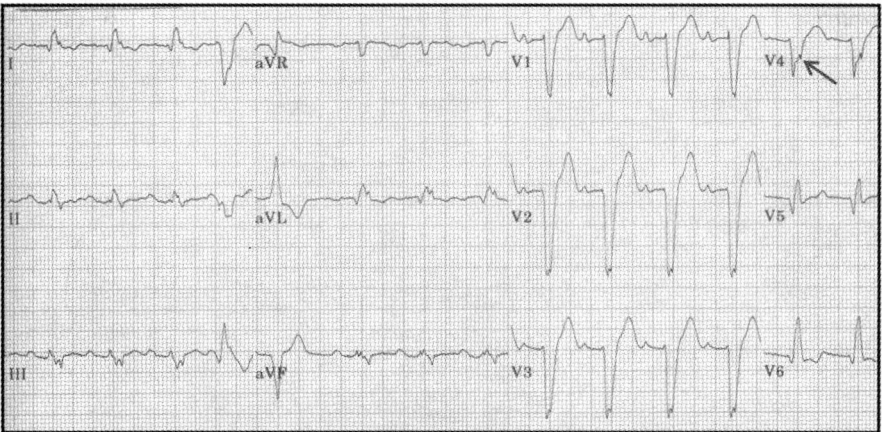

图 9 - 17

9.4　Non-ST elevation MI（NSTEMI）

- ECG changes may be minimal, or may show only T wave inversion, or may show ST segment depression with or without T wave inversion.
- Although it is tempting to localize the non-Q MI by the particular leads showing ST – T changes, this is probably only valid for the ST segment elevation MI's（STEMI）
  - Evolving ST – T changes may include any of the following patterns：
  - · ST segment depression in 2 or more leads（this carries the worse prognosis）
  - · Symmetrical T wave inversion only（this carries a better prognosis）
  - · Combinations of above changes
  - · OR the ECG may remain normal or only show minimal change（this has the best prognosis）

9.5　The Pseudoinfarcts

- These are ECG conditions that mimic myocardial infarction either by simulating pathologic Q or QS wavesor mimicking the typical ST – T changes of acute MI.
  - · WPW preexcitation（negative delta wave may mimic pathologic Q waves；see the ECG illustrated in Fig. 9 – 18. This is an interesting ECG with intermittent WPW preexcitation. The WPW pattern is seen on the first half of the ECG, but disappeared when the precordial leads V1 – 6 were recorded. Note the deep Q and QS waves in leads Ⅱ, Ⅲ, and aVF. These are not really Q waves but negative（down-going）delta waves. Note also the slurred upstroke of the QRS complex in leads Ⅰ, and the first half of the V5 rhythm strip（bottom channel）. In the 2nd half of the ECG tracing the "pseudo" Q waves in the lead Ⅱ rhythm strip disappear and a qR wave QRS complex appears indicating the return of normal conduction through the ventricles. Also the delta wave in lead V5 goes away on the bottom channel during the 2nd half of the ECG. Finally, the PR interval is also shorter during the 1st half of the ECG when preexcitation is occurring.

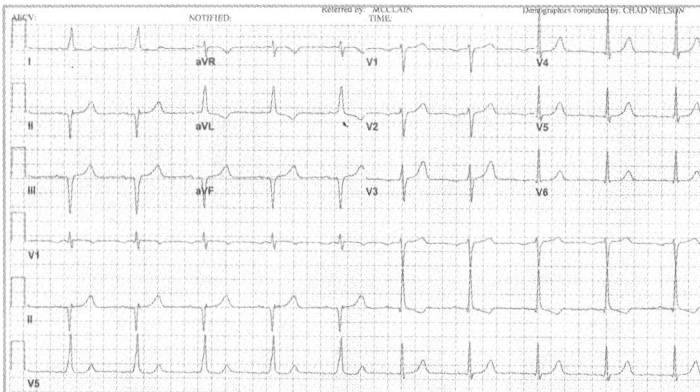

Intermittent WPW Preexcitation（1st half of ECG）with pseudo Q-waves Ⅱ, Ⅲ, aVF

Fig. 9 – 18

9.4 非 ST 段抬高型心肌梗死（NSTEMI）

- 心电图变化可能很小，也可能只显示 T 波倒置，或者可能显示 ST 段压低有或没有 T 波倒置。
- 虽然通过 ST－T 变化去给非 Q 波型心肌梗死定位很有诱惑，但是这可能只对定位 ST 段抬高型心肌梗死（STEMI）有效。
- ST－T 变化演变可能包括下列模式：
- · ST 段压低出现在 2 个或以上导联（这会带来预后不好）。
- · 只有 T 波呈对称型倒置（这会带来好的预后）。
- · 以上两者都有。
- · 或者心电图可以保留正常或仅有很小的改变（这个预后最好）。

9.5 假梗死

- 有些心电图模拟心肌梗死的心电图表现，通过模拟病理性 Q 波或 QS 波，或模仿急性心肌梗死典型 ST－T 改变。
- **WPW 预激综合征**（负 delta 波可能模仿病理性 Q 波，见图 9－18。这是一个有趣的心电图，表现为间歇性 WPW 预激。WPW 模式出现在心电图前半部，但当描记到胸前导联 V1～V6 时消失了。注意 Ⅱ，Ⅲ 和 aVF 有较深的 QS 波，没有真正的 Q 波，而是负的向下的 delta 波。也要注意 Ⅰ 导联 QRS 升支切迹，见最下面 V5 导联的前半部。在心电图后半部分 Ⅱ 导联的"假"Q 波消失，qR 波和 QRS 波群形态提示通过心室的传导恢复正常。后半段心电图下面 V5 导联的 delta 波也消失了。最后一点，心电图前半段当 WPW 预激发作时 PR 也短。

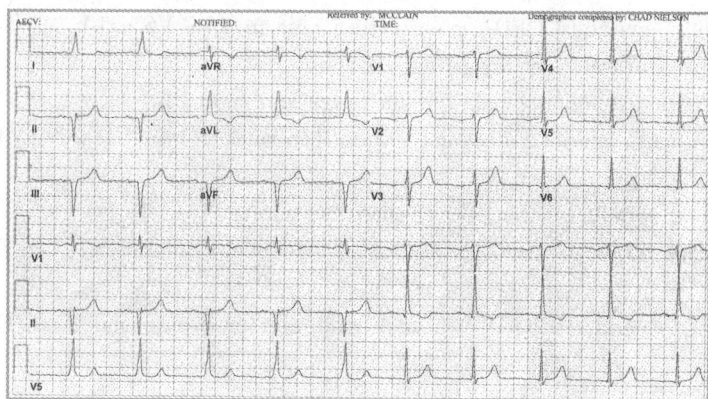

间歇性 WPW 预激（前半部 ECG）Ⅱ，Ⅲ，aVF 假 Q 波

图 9－18

· IHSS (septal hypertrophy may make normal septal Q waves "fatter" thereby mimicking pathologic Q waves)

· LVH (may have QS pattern or poor R wave progression in leads V1 – V3

· RVH (tall R waves in V1 or V2 may mimic true posterior MI)

· Complete or incomplete LBBB (QS waves or poor R wave progression in leads V1 – V3)

· Pneumothorax (loss of right precordial R waves)

· Pulmonary emphysema and cor pulmonale (loss of R waves V1 – 3 and/or inferior Q waves with right axis deviation)

· Left anterior fascicular block (may see small q-waves in anterior chest leads)

· Acute pericarditis (the ST segment elevation may mimic acute transmural injury)

· Central nervous system disease (may mimic non-Q wave MI by causing diffuse ST – T wave changes)

9.6 Miscellaneous Abnormalities of the QRS Complex in the differential diagnosis of MI

● Poor R Wave Progression – arbitrarily defined as small, or absent r-waves in leads V1 – V3 (R <2mm, plus R/S ratio V4 <1). Differential diagnosis includes:

· Normal variant (if the rest of the ECG is normal; frequently seen in women due to inaccurate precordial lead placement

· LVH (look for voltage criteria and ST – T changes of LV "strain")

· Complete or incomplete LBBB (also see increased QRS duration)

· Left anterior fascicular block (should see LAD $\geqslant$ – 45° in frontal plane)

· Anterior or anteroseptal MI (look for evolving ST – T changes)

· Emphysema and COPD (look for R/S ratio in V5 – V6 <1)

· Diffuse infiltrative or myopathic processes

· WPW preexcitation (look fordelta waves and short PR)

● Prominent Anterior Forces-defined as R/S ratio >1 in V1 or V2. Differential diagnosis includes:

· Normal variant (if the ECG is otherwise normal)

· True posterior MI (look for additional evidence of inferior MI; see Example 4, P150)

· RVH (should see RAD in frontal plane and/or P-pulmonale; see Example 2, P148)

· Complete or incomplete RBBB (look for rSR′ in V1)

· WPW preexcitation (look fordelta waves, short PR)

· Left septal fascicular block (not a universally accepted entity-but strong evidence exists for this)

- IHSS(间隔肥大可能使正常间隔 Q 波变"胖",从而像病理性 Q 波)。
- LVH(V1 ~ V3 导联可能有 QS 型即 R 波发展不良)。
- RVH(V1 和 V2 高 R 波可能像正后壁心肌梗死)。
- 完全或不完全的 LBBB(V1 ~ V3 导联可能有 QS 型,即 R 波发展不良)。
- 气胸(失去右心前区导联的 R 波)。
- 肺气肿和肺心病(R 波 V1 ~ V3 丢失和(或)下壁 Q 波与右轴右偏)。
- 左前分支阻滞(前胸导联可以看到小 q 波)。
- 急性心包炎(ST 段抬高可能像急性透壁的损伤)。
- 中枢神经系统疾病(可能模仿非 Q 波型心肌梗死导致弥漫性 ST – T 波变化)。

9.6 心肌梗死鉴别诊断中的各种复杂的 QRS 波群

● **R 波发展不良**:在 V1 ~ V3 导联中(R < 2 mm,再加上 V4 R/S 比值 < 1)定义为小 r,或无 r 波的情况。鉴别诊断包括:

- 正常变异(如果静息心电图正常,经常出现在女性,常由于不准确的心前导联位置)。
- LVH(寻找电压标准和左心室"压力负荷"的 ST – T 改变)。
- 完全或不完全的 LBBB(也可看到增加了 QRS 时间)。
- 左前分支阻滞(额面电轴左偏 ≥ – 45°)。
- 前壁或前间壁心肌梗死(寻找 ST – T 改变的演变)。
- 肺气肿和慢性阻塞性肺疾病(R/S V5 ~ V6 < 1)。
- 弥漫性浸润性肌病进展。
- WPW 预激(找 delta 波和短的 PR)。

● **明显向前的向量**:定义为 V1 或 V2 导联 R/S > 1。鉴别诊断包括:

- 正常变异(如果 ECG 正常)。
- 正后壁心肌梗死(注意同时有没有下壁心肌梗死的证据;见例 4,P151)。
- RVH(应见到额面电轴右偏和(或)肺性 P 波;见例 2,P149)。
- 完全性或不完全性 RBBB(rSR′ V1)。
- WPW 预激(delta 波,短 PR)。
- 左间隔支阻滞(实质上没有被广泛认同,但存在强有力的证据)。

10　ST Segment Abnormalities

General Introduction to ST, T, and U wave abnormalities

● Basic Concept: the specificity of ST – T and U wave abnormalities is determined more by the clinical circumstances in which the ECG changes are found than by the particular changes themselves. Thus the term, nonspecific ST – T wave abnormalities, is frequently used for ST segment depression and T wave abnormalities when the clinical data are not available to correlate with the ECG findings. This does not mean that the ECG changes are unimportant! It is the responsibility of the clinician providing care for the patient to ascertain the importance of the ECG findings.

● Factors affecting the ST – T and U wave configuration include:

· Intrinsic myocardial disease (e. g. , myocarditis, ischemia, infarction, infiltrative or myopathic processes)

· Drugs (e. g. , digoxin, antiarrhythmics, tricyclics, and many others)

· Electrolyte abnormalities of potassium, magnesium, and calcium

· Neurogenic factors (e. g. , stroke, CNS hemorrhage, head trauma, brain tumor, etc.)

· Metabolic factors (e. g. , hypoglycemia, hyperventilation)

· Atrial repolarization (e. g. , at fast heart rates the end of the atrial T wave may pull down the beginning of the ST segment; this is not a true ST segment change)

· Genetic abnormalities of channel membrane proteins, calledchannelopathies. Examples include hereditary long QT syndromes, and Brugada Syndrome.

● Secondary ST – T wave changes are the result of alterations in the sequence of ventricular depolarization (e. g. , bundle branch blocks, WPW preexcitation and ventricular ectopic beats or paced beats). These changes are not abnormalities; they are appropriate in the setting of altered ventricular activation sequence. ST – T wave changes are called primary if they are independent of the sequence of ventricular depolarization (e. g. , ischemic ST changes, electrolyte abnormalities, drug effects, etc.). These changes are repolarization abnormalities.

10　ST 段异常

ST 段，T 波和 U 波异常的一般概念

- **基本概念**：特异性 ST – T 和 U 波异常是由临床实践中发现心电图变化来决定的，而不是本身特有的那些变化。因此**非特异性 ST – T 波异常**这个术语通常指 ST 段压低和 T 波异常，而且用于临床资料不能有效提供与这些心电图表现的相关性时，但这不意味心电图变化不重要！**负责地为患者提供明确的重要的心电图结果是一个临床医生的责任。**

- 影响 ST – T 和 U 形态的因素包括：
- · 内在心肌疾病（如心肌炎、缺血、梗死、活动的浸润性心肌病）
- · 抗心律失常药物（如地高辛，三环类抗抑郁药和许多其他的药）
- · 电解质异常（钾，镁，钙）
- · 神经源性因素［例如脑卒中、中枢神经系统（CNS）出血、脑外伤、脑肿瘤等）］
- · 代谢因素（例如低血糖，换气过度）
- · 心房复极化（例如，在心率快时心房 T 波结束可能将 ST 段的起始部下拉，这不是一个真正的 ST 段变化）
- · 通道膜蛋白的基因异常，称为**通道病**。例如遗传性长 QT 综合征和 Brugada 综合征。

- **继发性 ST – T 改变**是心室除极顺序改变的结果（例如，束支阻滞，WPW 综合征和心室异位搏动或起搏器起搏）。这些变化不是异常，他们是心室激动顺序改变导致的适当的变化。如果 ST – T 改变不是由于心室去极化的顺序变化引起的，而是心肌本身有问题（如缺血、电解质异常，药物作用等），则称**原发性 ST – T 改变**。这些变化是复极化的异常。

10.1 Differential Diagnosis of ST Segment Elevation

Normal Variant "Early Repolarization Pattern" (ST segments are usually concave upwards, ending with symmetrical, large, upright T waves)

"Early Repolarization": note high take off of the ST segment in leads V4 – 6; ST segment elevation in V2 – 3 is generally seen in most normal ECG's; the ST elevation in V2 – 6 is concave upwards, another characteristic of this normal variant. This pattern is especially common in young, male athletes.

10.1.1 Ischemic Heart Disease (usually convex upwards, or straightened ST segment)

This is the result of transmural myocardial ischemia after total coronary occlusion.

Example 1: Acute anterior transmural injury – anteroseptal MI

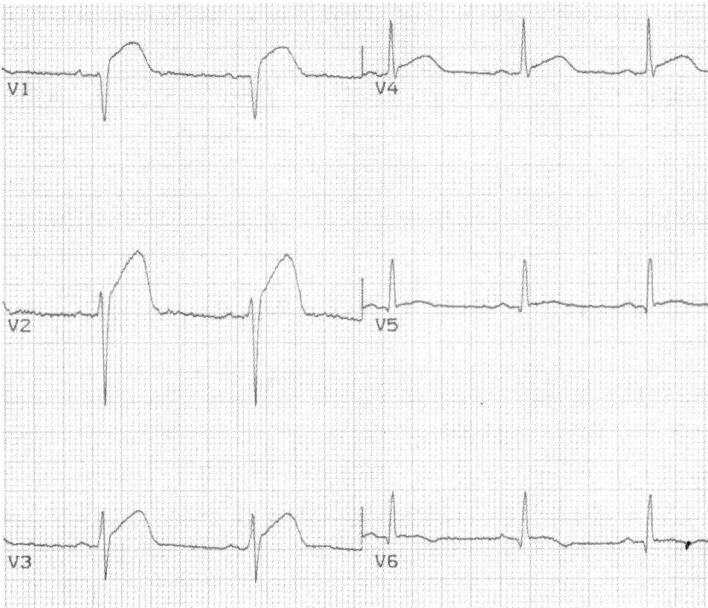

Fig. 10 – 1

• Note: Persistent ST elevation longafter an acute MI suggests failure of reperfusion, a ventricular aneurysm, or an akinetic scar resulting from a healed MI.

• Reversible ST elevation may also be seen as a manifestation of Prinzmetal's (or "variant") angina which is caused by transient coronary artery spasm. Coronary spasm can also occur as a result of cocaine overdose.

• ST elevation during exercise ECG testing suggests an extremely tight coronary artery stenosis or transient spasm (transmural ischemia).

10.1 ST 段抬高的鉴别诊断

正常变异："早期复极化模式"（ST 段通常凹面向上，有对称的、大的、直立的 T 波）。

"早期复极化"：注意 V4 ~ V6 的 ST 段起点高，V2 ~ V3 的 ST 段抬高通常在大多数正常心电图中也可以见到的；V2 ~ V6 的 ST 段是凹面向上抬高，这是正常变异的特点。这种模式的另一个特点是常见于年轻人，男运动员。

10.1.1 缺血性心脏病（ST 段抬高通常凸面向上，或变直的 ST 段）

这是由于冠状动脉完全闭塞导致的透壁性心肌缺血的结果。

例 1：急性前壁透壁性损伤：前间隔心肌梗死。

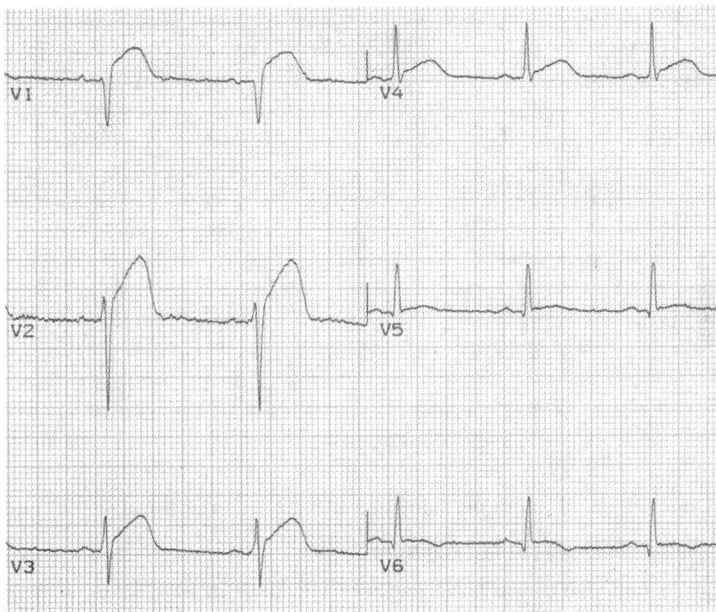

图 10 - 1

● 注意：急性心肌梗死后 ST 段长时间的持续抬高提示再灌注失败，室壁瘤形成，或来自于心肌梗死愈合形成的无收缩功能的瘢痕。

● 可逆的 ST 抬高见于变异型心绞痛，是由一过性冠状动脉痉挛所致。冠状动脉痉挛也可以产生于可卡因过量。

● 运动试验中 ST 抬高提示严重的冠状动脉狭窄或一过性冠状动脉痉挛（透壁性心肌缺血）。

10.1.2 Acute Pericarditis

- Concave upwards ST elevation in most leads except aVR
- No reciprocal ST segment depression (except in lead aVR)
- Unlike "early repolarization", T waves are usually lower in amplitude, and heart rate is usually increased.
- May see PR segment depression, a manifestation of atrial injury

Example 2: Post-op pericarditis; note diffuse, concave-upwards ST elevation, HR 100 bpm, PR segment depression in leads Ⅰ, V2, V3; PR segment elevation is seen in aVR.

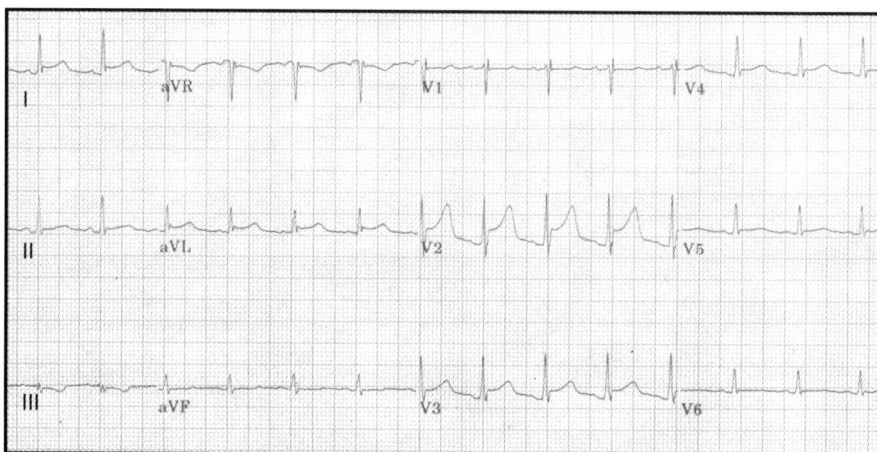

Fig. 10 - 2

The ECG changes of acute pericarditis evolve over time through the following stages (not all stages are seen in every patient):

- Stage Ⅰ: concave upwards ST segment elevation in most leads with reciprocal ST segment depression in aVR. During this stage there is also atrial injury represented by PR segment depression in many leads and PR segment elevation in aVR (see above example 2).
- Stage Ⅱ: resolution of ST segment and PR segment changes
- Stage Ⅲ: diffuse T wave inversion in many leads
- Stage Ⅳ: resolution of the T wave changes or persistent T wave inversion (chronic pericarditis)

10.1.2　急性心包炎

- 除了 aVR 外大多数导联 ST 段凹面向上抬高。
- 没有对应的导联 ST 段压低（除外 aVR）。
- 与"早期复极"不同的是，T 波振幅通常较低，心率通常是增加的。。
- 可能会看到 PR 段压低，心房损伤的表现。

例 2：术后心包炎；弥散的，ST 段凹面向上抬高，HR 100 次/min，Ⅰ、V2、V3 导联 PR 段压低；aVR 导联 PR 段抬高。

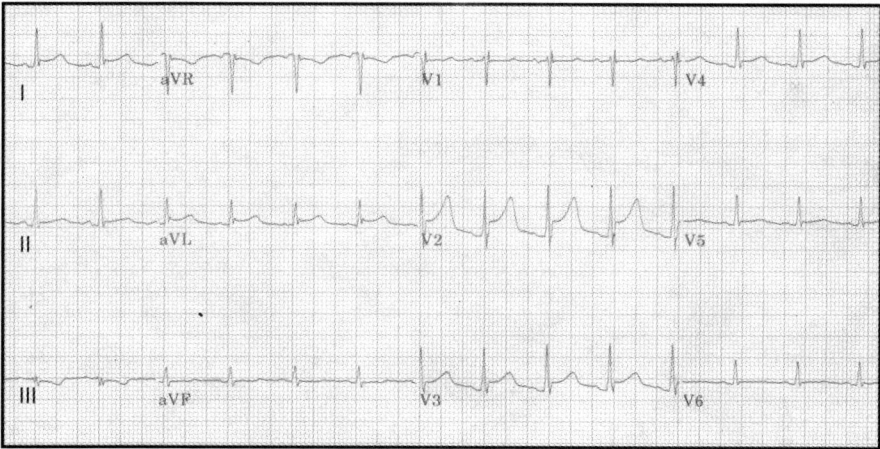

图 10 - 2

急性心包炎的心电图改变随时间推移而发展，包括下列各阶段（不是所有的阶段都出现在每一个患者）：

- 第一阶段：凹面向上 ST 段在大多数导联抬高，而对应导联 aVR 的 ST 段压低。在这个阶段也存在心房损伤表现在许多导联 PR 段压低而 aVR 导联 PR 段抬高（见例 2）。
- 第二阶段：ST 段和 PR 段的变化恢复。
- 第三阶段：许多导联弥漫性 T 波倒置。
- 第四阶段：T 波变化或持续 T 波倒置（慢性心包炎）。

10.1.3　Hypothermia

In this interesting condition the onset of the ST segment (called the J-point) turns into a wider J-wave as a result of increased transmural dispersion of ventricular repolarization. The ECG in Fig. 10 – 3 illustrates these prominent "J-Waves" following most of the QRS complexes (also called "Osborn" waves). This homeless person was found comatose in December outside in a park. Note also atrial fibrillation.

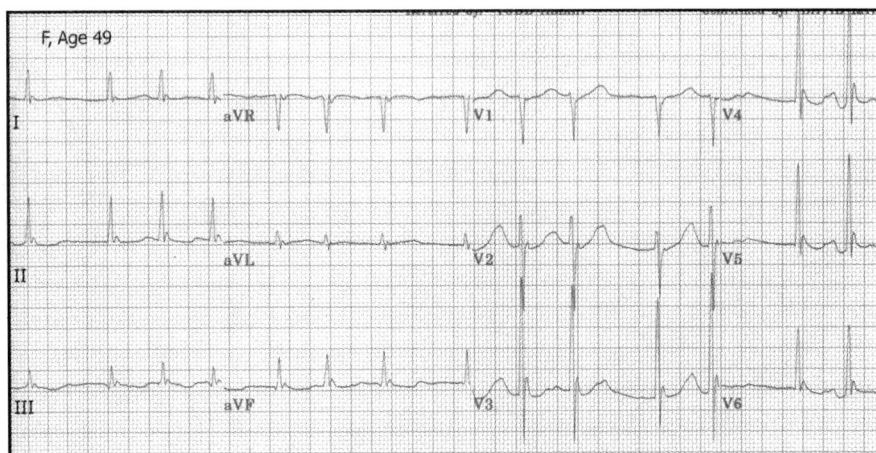

Hypothermia and Atrial Fibrillation

Fig. 10 – 3

10.1.4　Other Causes or ST segment elevation

- Left ventricular hypertrophy (seen in right precordial leads with large S-waves)
- Left bundle branch block (seen in right precordial leads with large S-waves)
- Advanced hyperkalemia (seen in multiple ECG leads with widened QRS complexes)

10.2　Differential Diagnosis of ST Segment Depression

10.2.1　Subendocardial ischemia

Subendocardial ischemia is the most common expression of ischemia during exercise ECG testing and is manifested as horizontal or downsloping ST depression mainly in the lateral precordial leads. The progression of these changes is illustrated in Fig. 10 – 4. Transmural ischemia is manifested by ST elevation. The leads showing the ST elevation often point to a critical lesion (or spasm) in a particular coronary artery.

10.1.3 体温过低

有趣的情况是 ST 段起始部(称为 J 点)变成了一个宽的 J 波,这是由于增加了心室复极化的透壁性分散的结果。图 10-3 的心电图显示了大多数 QRS 后的这些明显的"J 波"(也称为"Osborn"波)。一个冬季的 12 月份,这个无家可归的人被发现昏迷在公园外,还要注意心房纤颤。

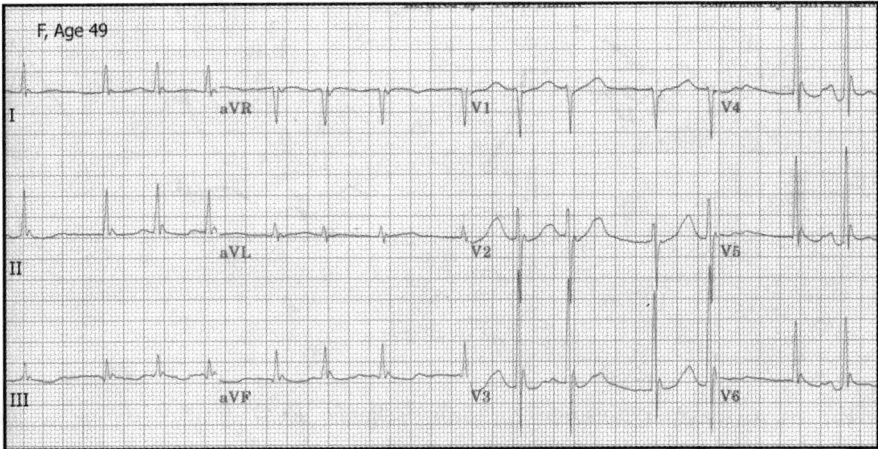

低体温症和心房纤颤

图 10-3

10.1.4 其他原因或 ST 段抬高

- 左心室肥大(见右心前区的导联伴有大 S 波)
- 左束支阻滞(见右心前区导联的大 S 波)
- 严重的血钾过高(在多个心电图导联可见宽大的 QRS 波)

10.2 ST 段压低的鉴别诊断

10.2.1 心内膜下心肌缺血

心内膜下心肌缺血是运动试验心电图最常见的缺血表达,主要表现为侧壁胸前导联的 ST 段呈水平型或下斜型压低。图 10-4 描述了这些变化的进展。透壁的缺血表现为 ST 段抬高。抬高的这些导联指定了一个特定的冠状动脉——那个危险病变或(痉挛)的部位。

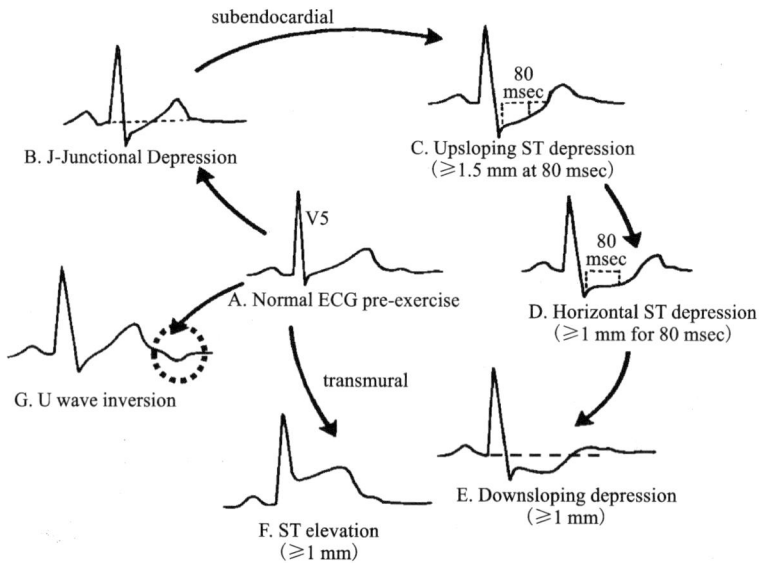

Fig. 10 – 4

The above diagram illustrates possible ischemic ECG changes during treadmill exercise testing as seen in lead V5; this is the best lead for identifying subendocardial ischemia as demonstrated by the sequence C-D-E.

A. Normal V5 ECG at rest before exercise (note normal ST – T and U waves)

B. J-junctional ST depression due to increased HR (this is not an ischemic change)

C. Early subendocardial ischemia (more J-junctional depression, slowly upsloping ST)

D. Horizontal ST segment depression (≥1mm, horizontal, lasting ≥80 ms)

E. Downsloping ST depression (usually seen during recovery from exercise as HR slows)

F. ST segment elevation (this is a manifestation oftransmural ischemia)

G. U-wave inversion (a very unusual manifestation of ischemia suggesting LAD or L-main disease). When seen, it occurs during recovery when HR slows down.

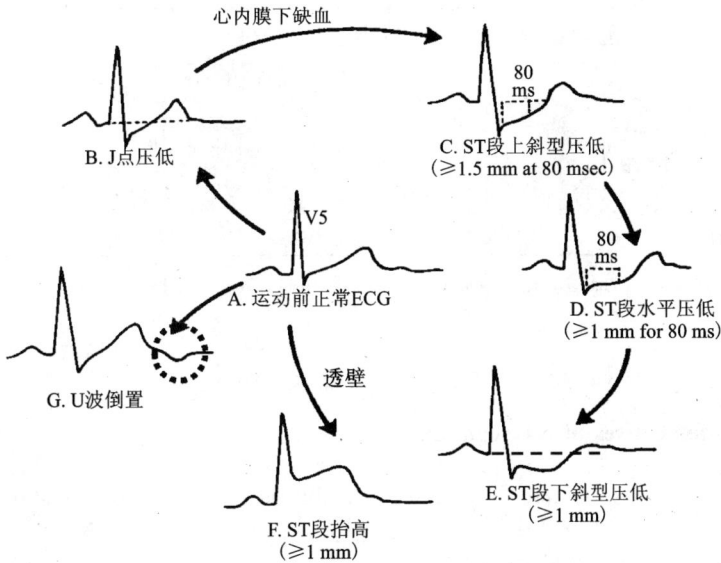

图 10 - 4

图 10 - 4 描述了踏车运动试验中 V5 导联见到的心电图缺血样改变，该导联是识别心内膜下缺血最好的导联，见图中 C - D - E 的系列变化。

A. 运动前正常 V5 静息心电图（注意正常 ST - T 和 U 波）

B. 因心率快，ST 起始部 J 点压低（这不是一个缺血性改变）

C. 早期心内膜下心肌缺血（J 进一步压低，缓慢的上斜形 ST 段）

D. 水平 ST 段压低（≥1 mm，水平，持续≥80 ms）

E. ST 段下斜形压低（通常在运动试验恢复心率放缓时见到）

F. ST 段抬高（这是透壁性缺血的表现）

G. U 波倒置（一个非常不寻常的缺血表现提示左前降支或左主干病变），当运动试验恢复心率放缓时可见到。

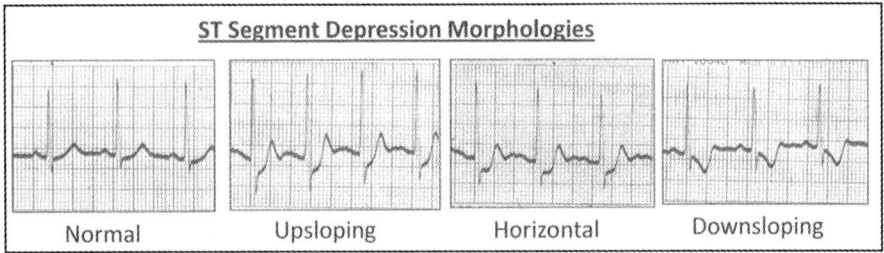

ST segment changes of subendocardial ischemia during exercise and recovery (V5)

Fig. 10 – 5

10. 2. 2　Other causes of ST segment depression

● Pseudo-ST-depression (wandering baseline artifact due to poor skin-electrode contact)

● Physiologic J-junctional depression with sinus tachycardia (most likely due to atrial repolarization and not a true ST change as seen in "B" in Fig. 10 – 4)

● Hyperventilation-induced ST segment depression (seen with anxiety)

● Non ST segment myocardial infarction (Non-STEMI)

● Reciprocal ST depression in STEMI (e. g. , ST depression in Ⅰ , aVL during an acute inferior STEMI)

● True posterior MI (ST depression in V1 – V3 reflects ST elevation in leads V8 – V9)

● "Strain" pattern of RVH (right precordial leads V1 – V3) and LVH (left precordial leads V5 – V6)

● Drugs (e. g. , digoxin)

● Electrolyte abnormalities (e. g. , hypokalemia)

● Neurogenic effects (in CNS disease)

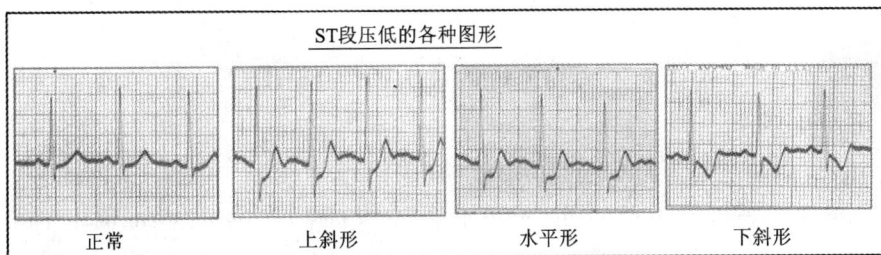

ST段压低的各种图形

| 正常 | 上斜形 | 水平形 | 下斜形 |

运动试验过程中心内膜下心肌缺血的 ST 段压低的各种形态（V5 导联）

图 10 – 5

10.2.2　ST 段压低的其他原因

● 假性 ST 压低（由于皮肤和电极接触不良导致人为的基线漂移）。

● 窦性心动过速时生理性 J 点降低（很可能由于心房复极引起而不是真正的 ST 改变，见图 10 – 4"B"）。

● 过度换气引起的 ST 段压低（见于焦虑）。

● 非 ST 段抬高型心肌梗死（Non-STEMI）。

● ST 段抬高型心肌梗死（STEMI）时对应导联 ST 段压低（如下壁 STEMI 时 Ⅰ，aVL 导联 ST 段压低）。

● 正后壁心肌梗死（V8 ~ V9 导联 ST 段抬高而 V1 ~ V3 导联 ST 段压低）。

● "负荷"型右心室肥大（右胸前导联 V1 ~ V3）和左心室肥大（左胸前导联 V5 ~ V6）。

● 药物（如地高辛）。

● 电解质紊乱（如低血钾）。

● 神经源性影响（如中枢神经系统疾病）。

11　T Wave Abnormalities

The T wave is the most labile wave in the ECG. T wave changes including low-amplitude T waves and abnormally inverted T waves may be the result of many cardiac and non-cardiac conditions. The normal T wave is usually in the same direction as the QRS except in the right precordial leads (see V1 – 3 in Fig. 11 – 1). The T wave in V1 may or may not be inverted, but usually from V2 on (in the adult person) the T waves are upright. Also, the normal T wave is asymmetric with the ascending half moving more slowly than the descending half. In the normal ECG, illustrated in Fig. 11 – 1, the T waves are always upright in leads Ⅰ, Ⅱ, V3 – V6, and always inverted in lead aVR. T waves in other leads are variable depending on the QRS axis and the age of the patient. Children and adolescents may have inverted T waves from V1 to V3.

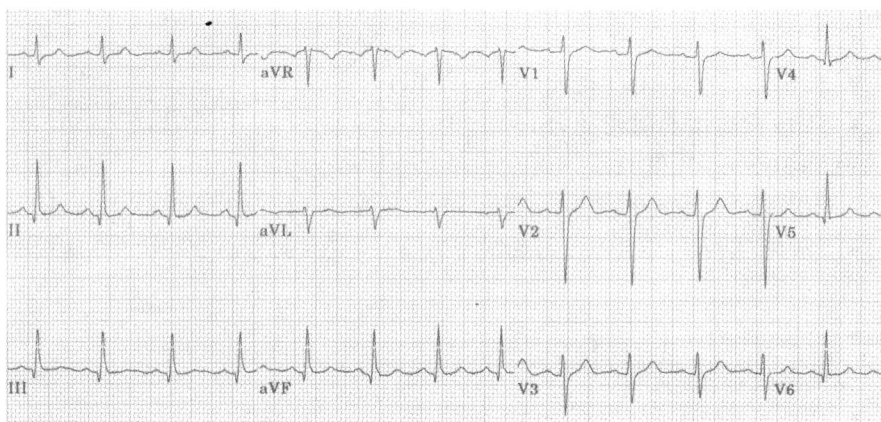

Normal ECG

Fig. 11 – 1

11.1　Differential Diagnosis of T Wave Inversion

- During the evolution of STEMI and NSTEMI. The precordial leads shown in Fig. 11 – 2 illustrate the evolved stage of an anterior MI after resolution of ST segment elevation:
- Subendocardial myocardial ischemia (e. g., during recovery from exercise testing)
- Subacute or healed pericarditis (see stages of pericarditis, P174)

11 T波异常

　　T波是心电图中最不稳定和容易变化的。T波改变包括低振幅T波和异常的T波倒置，这可能与心脏方面的原因有关，也可能与心脏外的因素有关。除右侧心前导联(V1~V3，见图11-1)外一般正常T波与QRS波方向一致。T波在V1导联可以是倒置的，也可以不是倒置的，但是在V2导联(成人)通常是直立的。而且，正常的T波是非对称的，升支运动慢于降支。图11-1的ECG描述了T波在Ⅰ，Ⅱ，V3~V6导联总是直立的，而在aVR导联总是倒置的。T波在其他导联的变化取决于QRS电轴以及患者的年龄。儿童和青少年可以有V1~V3的T波倒置。

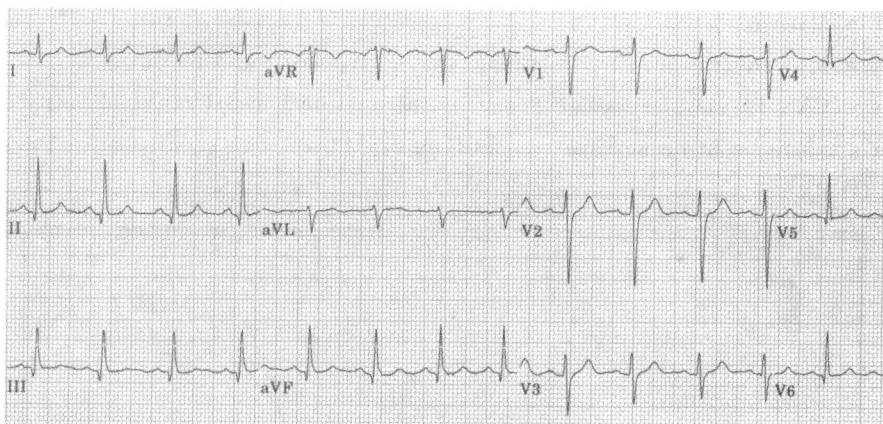

正常心电图

图11-1

11.1 T波倒置的鉴别诊断

　　● T波在STEMI和non-STEMI中的演变。图11-2是前壁心肌梗死胸前导联ST段抬高后的T波演变阶段。

　　● 心内膜下心肌缺血(如在运动试验恢复中)。

　　● 亚急性和愈合的心包炎(见P175心包炎的各阶段)。

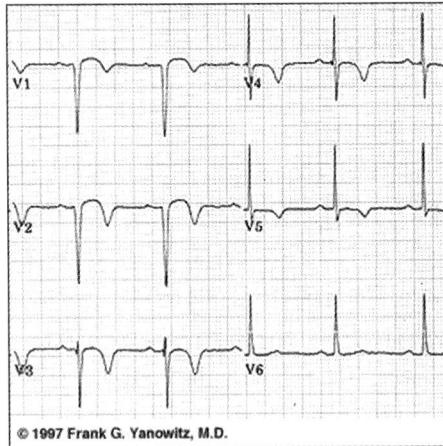

Fig. 11 – 2

- Myocarditis

- Myocardial contusion (from trauma; e. g. , steering wheel accident)

- CNS disease (neurogenic T wave changes) with long QT intervals (especially after a subarachnoid hemorrhage; see ECG in Fig. 11 – 3 with giant negative T waves and QT prolongation)

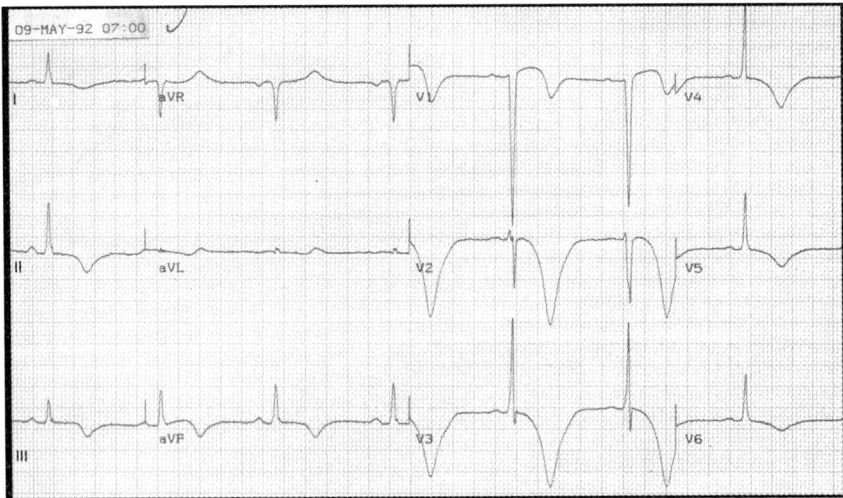

Giant Negative T waves

Fig. 11 – 3

- Idiopathic apical hypertrophy (a rare form of hypertrophic cardiomyopathy with giant negative T waves)

- Mitral valve prolapse (some cases)

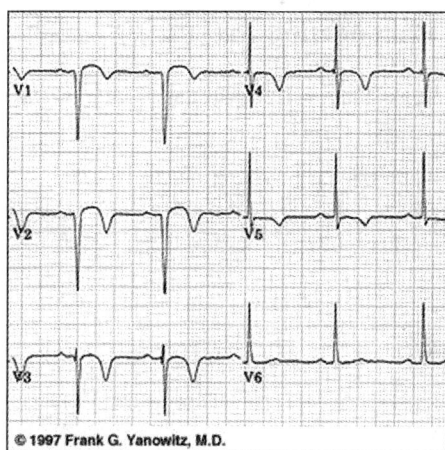

图 11 - 2

● 心肌炎。

● 心肌挫伤（来自创伤，如方向盘事故）。

● 中枢神经系统（神经源性 T 波改变）伴长 QT 间期（尤其是蛛网膜下隙出血之后；见图 11 - 3 心电图中巨大的倒置的 T 波伴有长 QT 间期）。

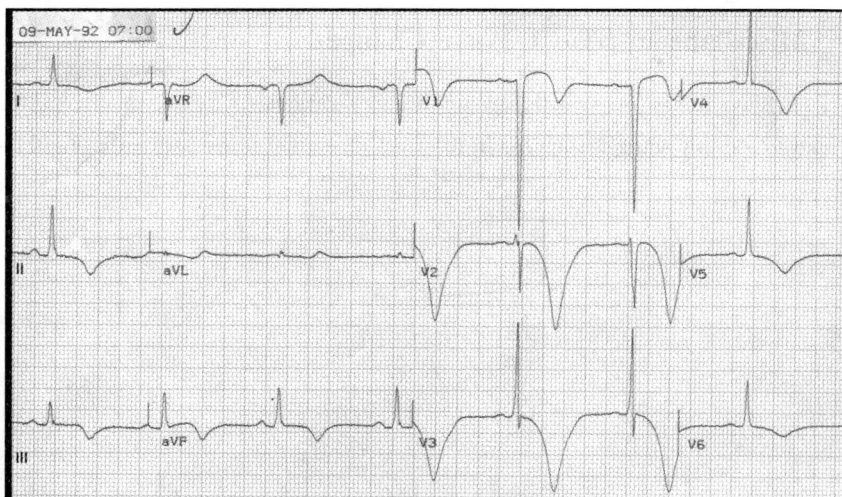

巨大倒置 T 波

图 11 - 3

● 特发性心尖肥厚型心肌病（一种罕见的肥厚型心肌病伴大的倒置 T 波）。

● 二尖瓣脱垂（某些病例）。

11.2 QT Interval Prolongation（see P34 for causes）

Example 1：Hereditary long QT syndrome（note the unusual bifid, humped T waves in V2 – V3）

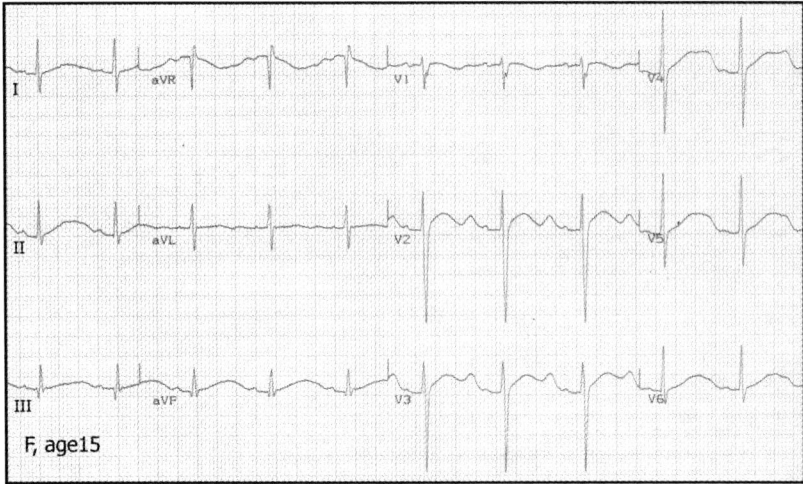

Fig. 11 – 4

11.3 Miscellaneous ST – T Wave Change

（1）Epsilon waves in Arrhythmogenic Right Ventricular Cardiomyopathy（ARVC）; these hard to see tiny squiggles appear in the right precordial leads（arrows in Fig. 11 –5）.

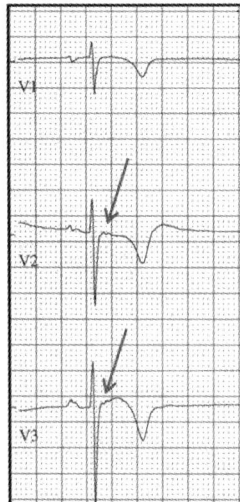

Fig. 11 – 5

11.2　QT 间期延长

了解 QT 间期延长的原因可参阅 P35 内容。

例 1：遗传性长 QT 间期综合征（注意 V2 ~ V3 导联那些不寻常的、分开的、隆起的 T 波）

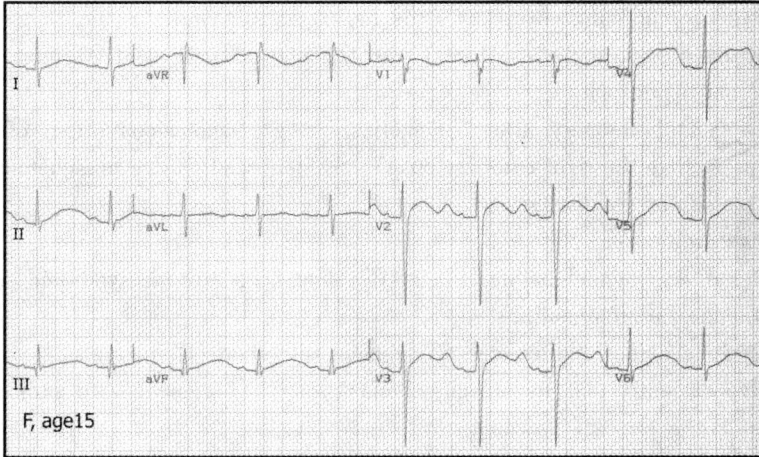

图 11 - 4

11.3　各种复杂的 ST - T 改变

（1）致心律失常型右心室心肌病（ARVC）可见 epsilon 波；这些很难看到的小线形波出现在右心前导联（图 11 - 5 箭头所示）。

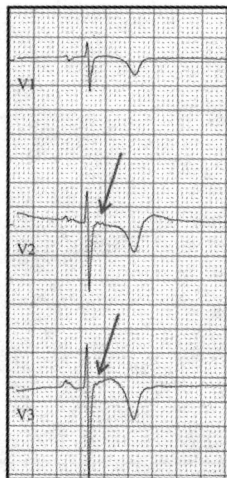

图 11 - 5

ARVC is a rare cause of sudden cardiac death in athletes. The disease usually involves the right ventricular outflow tract; normal myocardium is replaced by fatty infiltration and fibrosis. ECG manifestations include the very difficult to recognizeepsilon wave as well as right precordial T wave inversions (see the ECG in Fig. 11 −5).

(2) Other causes of sudden cardiac death in young athletes include:

● Hypertrophic cardiomyopathy (the most common cause in the U. S.). ECG findings in this disease include diffuse T wave inversions, prolonged QT intervals, and left ventricular hypertrophy.

● Congenital coronary artery anomalies (e. g. , anomalous origin of the left coronary artery from the right coronary cusp). Sudden death is due to ischemic events.

● Coronary artery disease

● Myocarditis

● Hereditary channelopathies (long QT, short QT, Brugada syndrome, et al)

(3) Electrolyte abnormalities

● Hypercalcemia (abbreviated ST segment with short QT intervals

● Hypocalcemia and hypomagnesaemia (long ST segment with prolonged QT intervals)

● Hyperkalemia (peaked T waves, prolonged QRS duration; see ECG below)

● Hypokalemia (usual triad of: ST depression, low T waves, and large U waves)

● Digoxin effect: scooped ST depression, low amplitude T waves, short QT intervals.

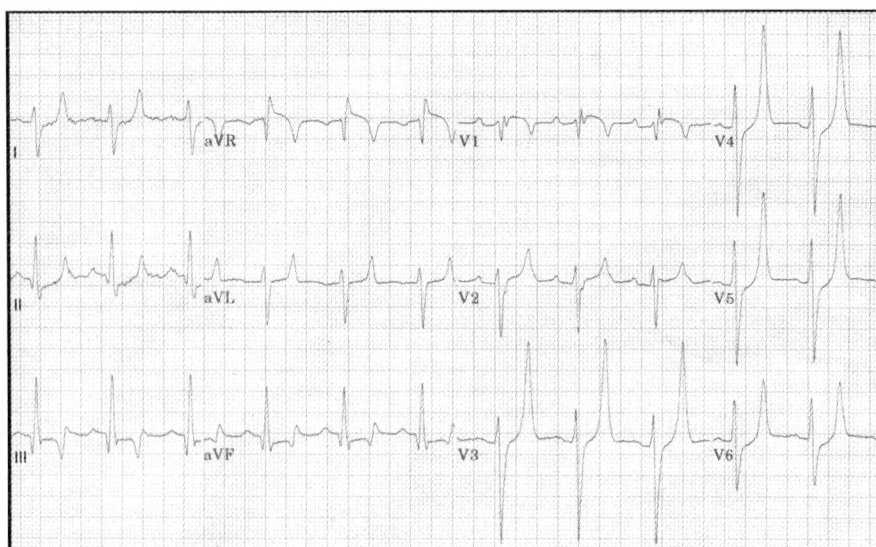

Hyperkalemia: tall, pointed, narrow T waves (avoid sitting on them!)

Fig. 11 −6

ARVC 是一种罕见的运动员心脏猝死的原因。这种疾病通常累及右心室流出道；正常心肌被脂肪浸润、纤维化所取代。心电图表现包括很难识别 epsilon 波以及右心前导联的 T 波倒置（图 11 – 5）。

（2）其他导致年轻运动员猝死的原因包括：

● 肥厚型心肌病（美国的最常见原因）。这种疾病的心电图表现包括弥漫性 T 波倒置，长 QT 间期，左心室肥大。

● 先天性冠状动脉异常（例如，左冠状动脉异常起源于右冠窦）。猝死是由于缺血性事件。

● 冠状动脉疾病。

● 心肌炎。

● 遗传性通道病（长 QT 间期，短 QT 间期，Brugada 综合征等）。

（3）电解质紊乱

● 高钙血症（缩短的 ST 段和 QT 间期）。

● 低钙血症和低镁血症（长 ST 段，长 QT 间隔）。

● 高钾血症（心电图 T 波高尖，QRS 时限延长，见下面心电图）。

● 低钾血症（常见三联征：ST 段压低、T 波低平和较大 U 波）。

● 地高辛效应：勺型 ST 段压低、T 波振幅低，短 QT 间期。

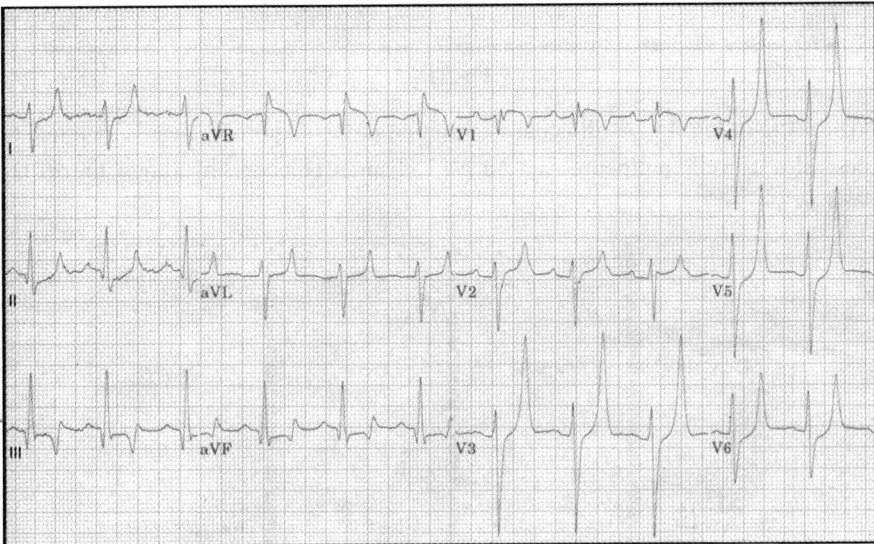

高钾血症：高，尖，窄的 T 波（不要坐在它们上面！）

图 11 – 6

（4）Brugada type ECG（seen in the hereditary Brugada syndrome and the acquired Brugada sign brought out by Na$^+$ channel blockers such as flecainide）; this is an unusual pattern of right precordial ST segment elevation with or without T wave inversion. An example is seen in the ECG in Fig. 11 − 7. Note that leads V1 and V2 might be confused with RBBB, but the QRS duration is not prolonged in other leads. Like the long QT syndrome, there is increased incidence of malignant arrhythmias and sudden cardiac death in this condition.

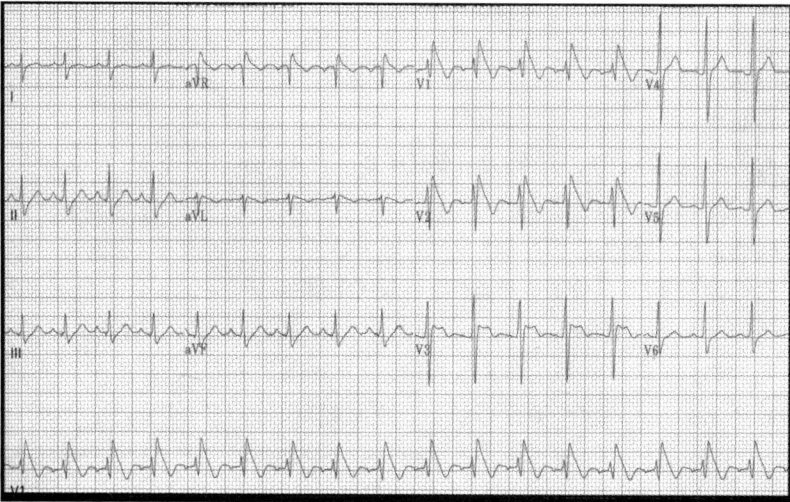

Fig. 11 −7

The ECG in Fig. 11 − 8 illustrates resolution of the acquired Brugada sign due to an overdose of a tricyclic antidepressant, a Na$^+$ channel blocker（by Day 4 the ECG has returned to normal）.

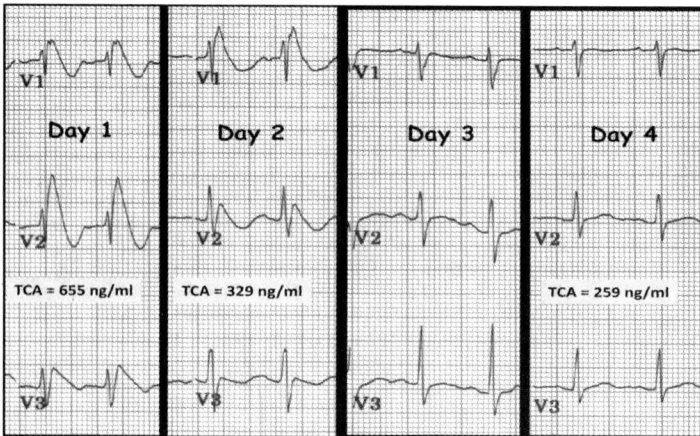

Fig. 11 −8

（4）Brugada 类型心电图（遗传性 Brugada 综合征和后天获得型 Brugada 征，后者由 Na⁺ 通道阻滞药，如氟卡尼等导致），这是一个不寻常的模式，心前导联的 ST 段抬高伴或不伴 T 波倒置。图 11－7 的心电图就是一个例子。注意，V1 和 V2 容易与 RBBB 混淆，但 QRS 时限在其他导联并不长。这种情况和长 QT 综合征一样会增加恶性心律失常和心脏猝死的发生率。

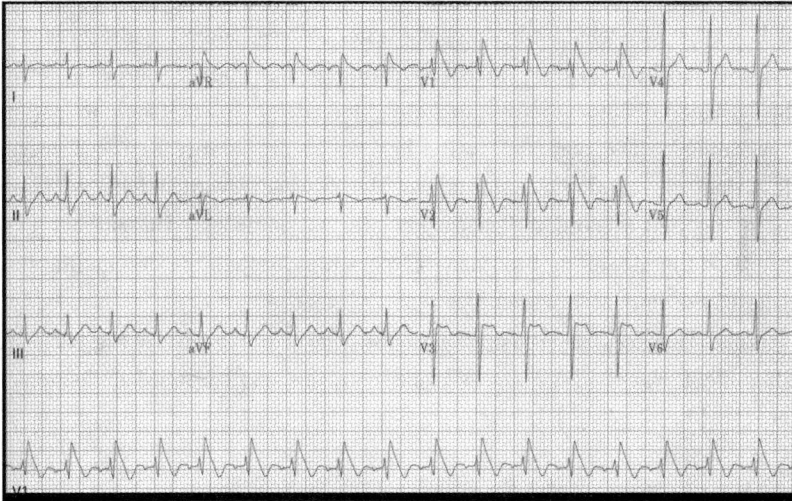

图 11－7

图 11－8 的心电图是一个服用了过量的三环类抗抑郁药（一种 Na⁺ 通道阻滞药）导致的获得性 Brugada 征（4 天心电图才恢复正常）。

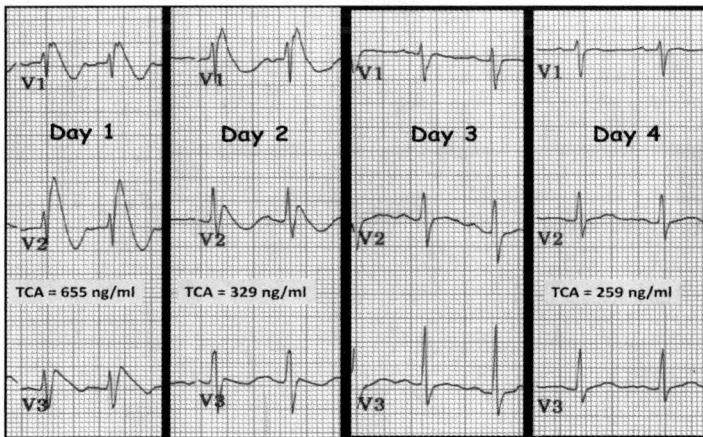

图 11－8

12 U Wave Abnormalities

The U wave is the only remaining enigma of the ECG, and probably not for long. The origin of the normal U wave is still in question, but many experts correlate abnormal U waves with electrophysiologic events called "after depolarizations" in the ventricular myocardium. These afterdepolarizations can be a source of arrhythmias caused by "triggered automaticity" including torsade de pointesseen in patients with long QT syndromes. The normal U wave has the same polarity as the T wave and is usually less than one-third the amplitude of the T wave. Normal U waves are usually best seen in the mid-precordial leads especially V2 and V3. The normal U wave is asymmetric with the ascending limb moving more rapidly than the descending limb (just the opposite of the normal T wave).

● Normal U waves are illustrated in the precordial leads in Fig. 12 – 1. Look closely after the T waves in V2 and V3 and note the small upward deflections. That's looking at "U" !!

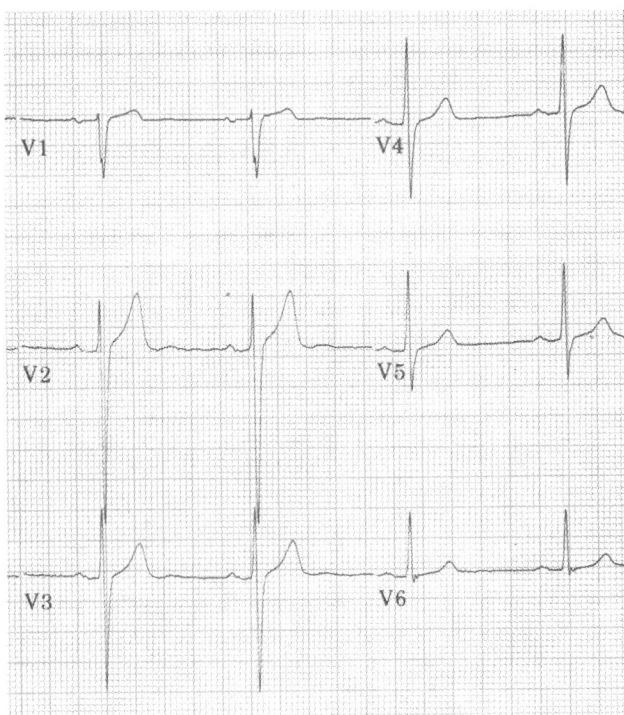

Fig. 12 – 1

12 U 波异常

U 波是唯一剩下的心电图的谜，而且可能不会持续太久。正常 U 波的起源仍然是个问题，但是许多专家将与电生理事件相关的异常 U 波称为心室心肌"后除极"。这些后除极就是"触发活动"引起心律失常的来源，包括在长 QT 间期综合征中所见到的**尖端扭转型室性心动过速**。正常 U 波极性与 T 波相同，振幅通常不到 T 波的三分之一。正常 U 波通常是中部心前导联特别是 V2 和 V3 最明显。正常 U 波是不对称的，升支速度高于降支(恰好与 T 波的相反)。

● 图 12－1 的心电图显示的是心前导联的正常 U 波。仔细看在 V2 和 V3 的 T 波后面的小直立波。你正在看的就是"U"波！！

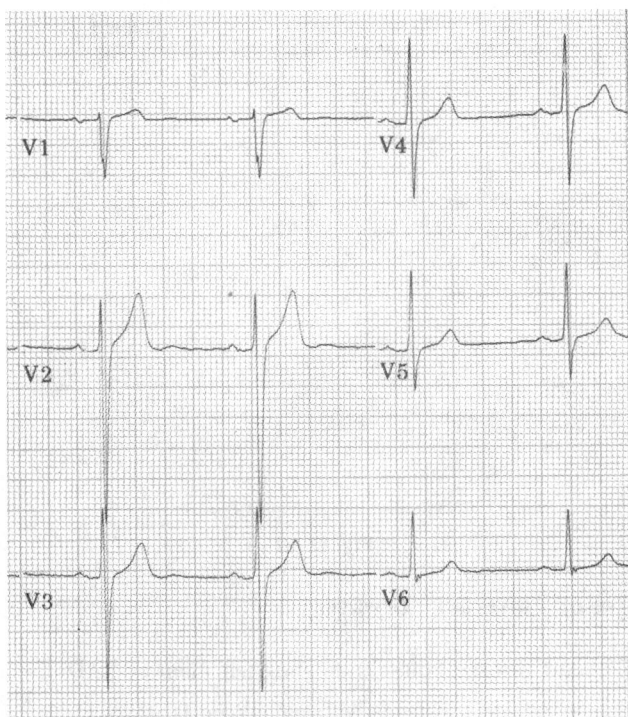

图 12－1

12.1 Differential Diagnosis of U Wave Abnormalities

12.1.1 Prominent upright U waves

• Sinus bradycardia accentuates normal U waves (this is normal)

• Hypokalemia (remember the triad of ST segment depression, low amplitude T waves, and prominent upright U waves)

• Various drugs including antiarrhythmics (e. g. , sotolol)

• LVH (may see prominent upright or inverted U waves in left precordial leads)

• CNS disease and other causes of long QT (T – U fusion waves); see ECG in Fig. 12 – 2.

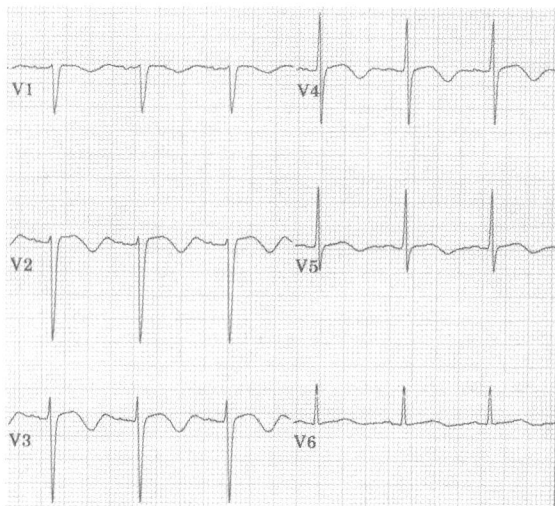

CNS disease with prominent U waves

Fig. 12 – 2

12.1.2 Negative or "inverted" U waves

(1)Ischemic heart disease (often indicating left main or LAD disease)

• Myocardial infarction (in leads with pathologic Q waves)

• During episode of acute ischemia (angina or exercise-induced ischemia; see diagram on P176)

• Post extrasystolic in patients with coronary heart disease

• During coronary artery spasm (Prinzmetal's angina)

• Left ventricular hypertrophy

12.1　U 波异常的鉴别诊断

12.1.1　明显直立的 U 波

- 窦性心动过缓突出正常 U 波(这是正常的)。
- 低钾血症(记住 ST 段的三联征：ST 压低、低振幅 T 波和明显直立的 U 波)。
- 各种药物包括抗心律失常药(例如索他洛尔)。
- LVH(可以看到明显的直立或倒置的 U 波在左心前导联)。
- 中枢神经系统疾病和其他原因的长 QT 间期(T–U 融合波)。请参阅图 12–2 的心电图。

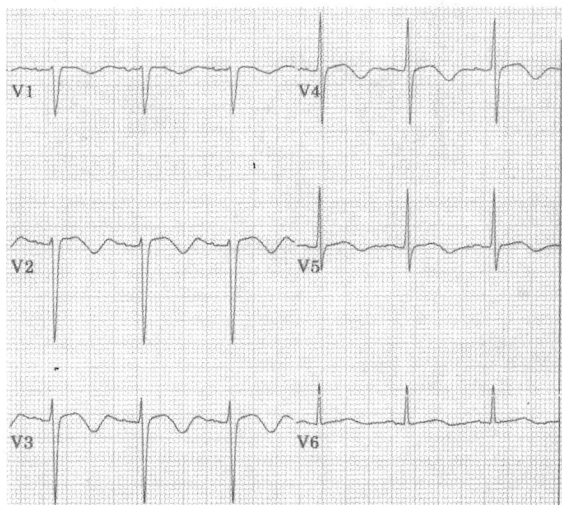

中枢神经系统疾病伴显著的 U 波

图 12–2

12.1.2　负的即"倒置"U 波

(1)缺血性心脏病(通常意味左主干或左前降支病变)
- 心肌梗死(有病理性 Q 波的导联)
- 急性缺血事件时(心绞痛或运动性缺血;见 P177 图示)
- 冠心病患者期外收缩后
- 冠状动脉痉挛(变异型心绞痛)
- 左心室肥大

（2）Nonischemic causes: some cases of LVH or RVH（usually in leads with prominent R waves）

• Some patients with LQTS（see Fig. 12 – 3: Lead V6 shows giant negative TU fusion wave in patient with LQTS; a prominent upright U wave is seen in Lead V1）

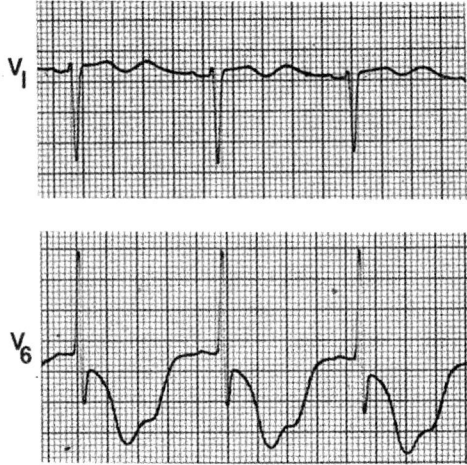

"U"-nbelievable

Fig. 12 – 3

（2）非缺血性因素：某些 LVH 或 RVH 的因素（通常表现在 R 波突出的导联）。

● 某些长 QT 间期综合征(LQTS)的患者（见图 12 - 3：患 LQTS 的患者，V6 导联可见大的负向的 TU 融合波；V1 导联可见某些直立的 U 波）。

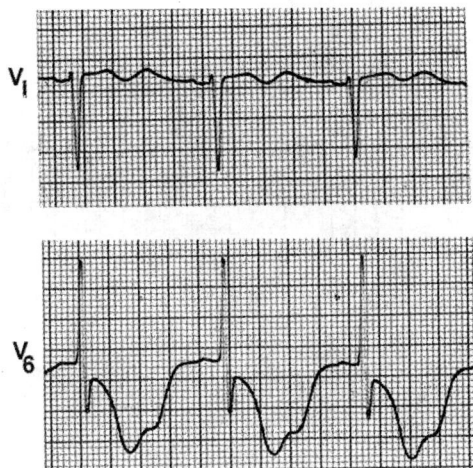

难以置信的"U"

图 12 - 3

习　题

1. 下面心电图的 **V1** 导联中宽大畸形的波（看样子很滑稽的波）诊断是什么？

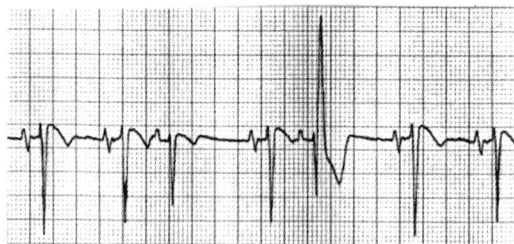

A. 房性期前收缩伴 LBBB 型差异性传导

B. 房性期前收缩伴 RBBB 型差异性传导

C. 来自右心室的室性期前收缩

D. 来自左心室的室性期前收缩

2. 下面 **V1** 导联的各 **QRS** 波群中"**F**"意味什么？

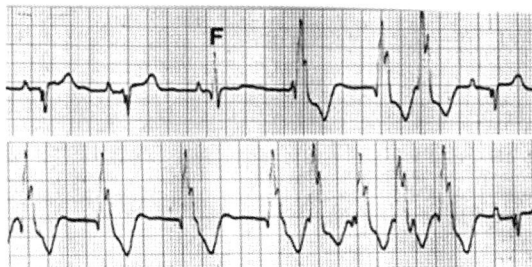

A. "F"是"看上去滑稽的波"

B. "F"是"夺获失败"，意味着窦 P 不能进入心室

C. "F"是"融合波"，如右心室期前收缩与窦性下传的 QRS 起始部融合

D. "F"是"融合波"，如左心室期前收缩与窦性下传的 QRS 起始部融合

3. 下面心电图 **V1** 中宽大的 **QRS** 节律的 **RR** 间期为什么不等？

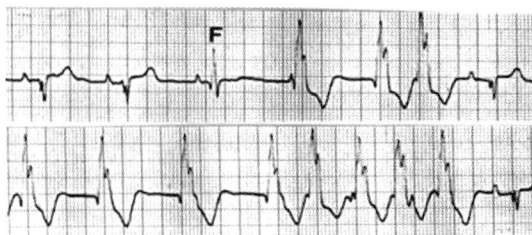

A. 这是室性心动过速伴间歇 2:1 传导阻滞

B. 这是阵发性心房纤颤与 RBBB 型差异性传导

C. 心室逸搏节奏与室性心动过速交替出现

D. 这是窦性心律伴心率相关性右束支传导阻滞

4. 下面心电图 V1 导联的条图除了正常窦性搏动外有 **4** 个畸形波(看上去滑稽),它们是什么?

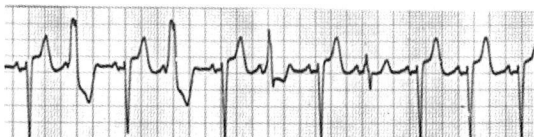

A. 它们是来自多个异位起搏点的室性期前收缩

B. 第 1 个宽大畸形是迟发室性期前收缩,其他 3 个是融合波

C. 间歇性 RBBB 型

D. 间歇性 WPW

5. 这个心电图 **V1** 的条图中是什么样的传导阻滞(如果有)?

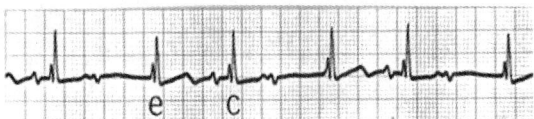

A. 1 度 AVB   B. 2 度 AVB

C. 3 度 AVB   D. 无 AVB;这是房室分离

6. 这个心电图 **V1** 的条图中"e"和"c"代表什么?

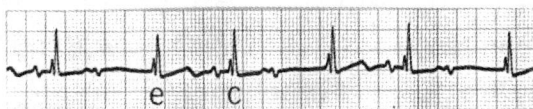

A. "e"代表 1 个未下传 P 的心室回声波,"c"窦性夺获

B. "e"是心室夺获,"c"是房性期前收缩

C. "e"是交界性逸搏,"c"代表房性期前收缩

D. "e"代表交界性逸搏;"c"代表窦性夺获

7. 这个心电图有点复杂的节律其实有一个非常简单的解释,是什么?

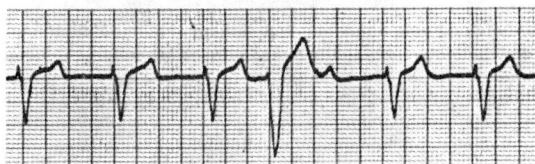

A. 交界性心律伴偶发室性期前收缩

B. 完全性 AVB

C. 窦性心律伴 1 度 AVB，偶发室性期前收缩

D. 交界性心律，房性期前收缩，以及未下传的房性期前收缩

8. 这个心电图 **V1** 导联的心电图条图有几个有趣的特点，在这个节律中是什么导致间歇产生？

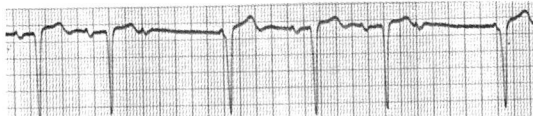

A. 2 度 AVB（Ⅰ型，文氏型）   B. 2 度 AVB（Ⅱ型，莫氏型）

C. 房性期前收缩未下传   D. 明显的窦性心律不齐

9. 这个 **V1** 导联的心电图条图有几个有趣的特点，是什么终止了间歇？

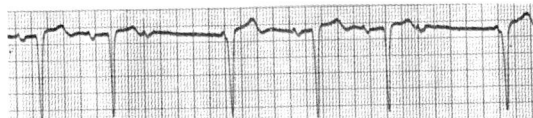

A. 被房性期前收缩重置的一个窦性搏动   B. 一个室性逸搏

C. 一个来自右心室的电子起搏器的起搏   D. 一个交界性逸搏

10. 这个心电图二联律诊断是什么？

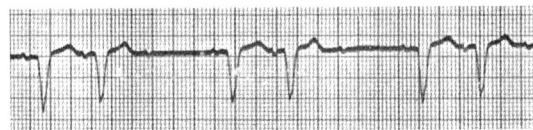

A. 2 度Ⅱ型 AVB（莫氏）   B. 未下传房性期前收缩后面跟随 2 个窦性搏动

C. 2 度Ⅰ型 AVB（文氏）   D. 窦房传出阻滞

11. 下面心电图中的 **QRS** 电轴是多少？

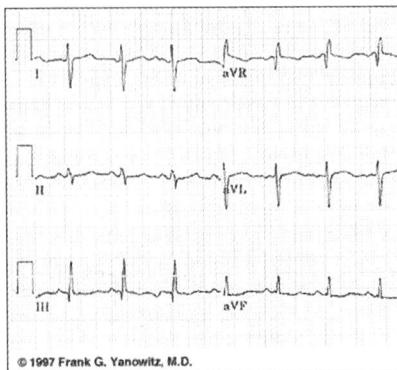

© 1997 Frank G. Yanowitz, M.D.

A. 无法确定   B. +90°   C. −30°

D. −45°   E. +150°

12. 确定下面心电图的 QRS 电轴是多少？

© 1997 Frank G. Yanowitz, M.D.

A. +90°   B. 无法确定   C. +30°

D. −30°   E. −150°

13. 什么是 QRS 电轴的正常范围？

A. 0～180°   B. 0～+90°   C. −30～+90°

D. −90～+90°   E. −90～+30°

14. 测量 V1 和 V2 导联的电流是什么方向？

A. 左向右   B. 向左前   C. 由前向后

D. 由上向下   E. 由内向外

15. 什么导联的电流方向和 I 导联相同？

A. aVF   B. II   C. III

D. V1   E. V6

16. 确定下列心电图的电轴是多少？

© 1997 Frank G. Yanowitz, M.D.

A. −60°   B. −45°   C. +60°

D. 无法确定   E. 0°

17. 确定下列心电图的电轴是多少？

© 1997 Frank G. Yanowitz, M.D.

A. −75°   B. −30°   C. 0°

D. +45°   E. 无法确定

18. 什么导联的电流方向是由上向下的？

A. I   B. aVF   C. aVL

D. V1   E. V6

19. 确定下列心电图的电轴是多少？

© 1997 Frank G. Yanowitz, M.D.

A. −15°   B. +15°   C. +60°

D. +105°   E. 无法确定

20. 确定下列心电图的电轴是多少？

© 1997 Frank G. Yanowitz, M.D.

A. −100° B. −30° C. +15°

D. +90° E. 无法确定

21. 下面心电图中 2 个箭头所指是什么心律失常？

A. 房性期前收缩

B. 室性期前收缩

C. 1 是房性期前收缩，2 是室性期前收缩

D. 阵发性室上性心动过速

22. 下面心电图中所见，是什么类型的心律失常？

A. 交界区期前收缩　　　　B. 频率依赖性束支传导阻滞

C. 房性期前收缩伴差异性传导　　D. 室性期前收缩

23. 下面心电图 2 个期前收缩的间歇是哪种？

Lead V₁

A. 完全性代偿间歇　　　　　　　B. 不完全性代偿间歇

C. 无间歇　　　　　　　　　　　D. 插入型间歇

E. 以上都不是

24. 说明下列心电图的心律失常是哪种？

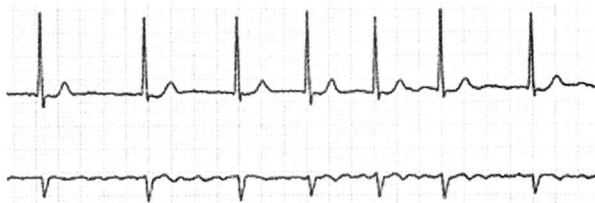

A. 交界性期前收缩　　　　　　　B. 心房扑动

C. 心房纤颤　　　　　　　　　　D. 房室结折返型心动过速

E. 加速性交界性心律

25. 下面心电图 2 个导联（Ⅲ，aVF）所见是什么？

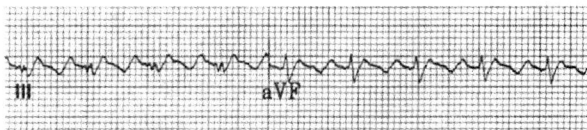

A. 窦性心动过速　　　　　　　　B. 阵发性室上性心动过速

C. 3 度 AVB　　　　　　　　　　D. 心房纤颤

E. 心房扑动 2：1 阻滞

26. 这个梯形图描述是哪种心律失常？

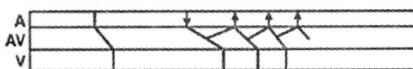

A. 窦性心动过速　　　　　　　　B. 房室结折返性心动过速

C. WPW 综合征　　　　　　　　　D. 频发房性期前收缩

E. 房性心动过速

27. 选择下列心电图的正确诊断：

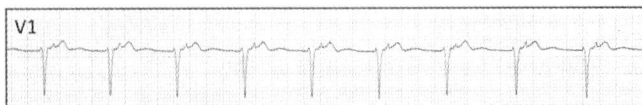

A. 正常窦性心律　　　　　　　　B. 心房纤颤

C. 窦性心动过速　　　　　　　　D. 交界性逸搏心律

E. 加速性交界性心律

28. 这个心律失常是什么?

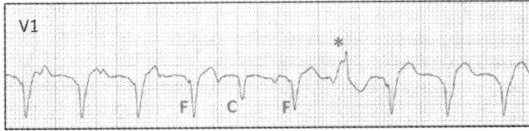

A. 室性心动过速
B. 室上性心动过速伴差异性传导
C. 加速性交界性心律
D. 加速性室性心律
E. 室性期前收缩二联律

29. 给下图作出正确的心电图诊断:

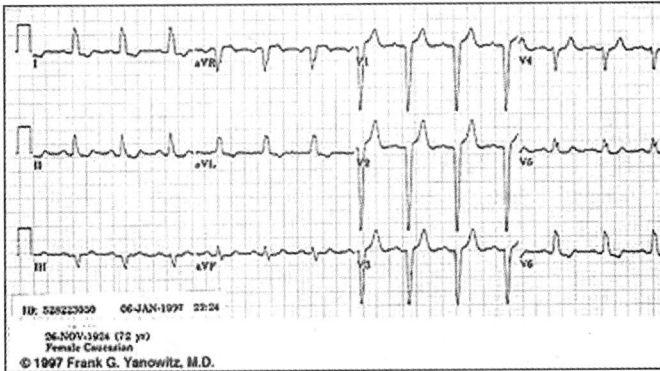

A. LBBB
B. RBBB
C. LAFB(左前分支阻滞)
D. RBBB + LAFB
E. RBBB + LPFB(左后分支阻滞)

30. 给下图作出正确的心电图诊断:

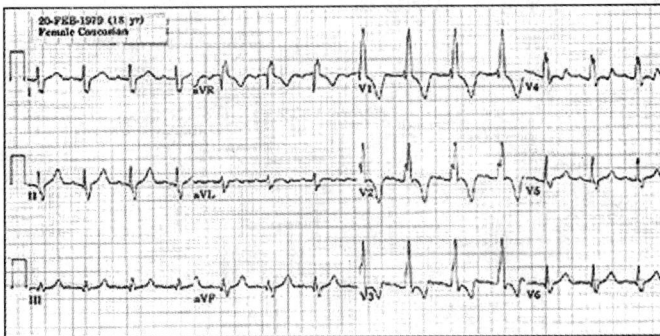

A. LBBB
B. RBBB
C. LAFB
D. RBBB + LAFB
E. RBBB + LPFB

31. 给下图作出正确的心电图诊断:

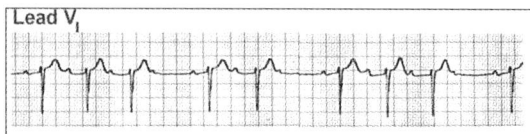

A. 1 度 AVB　　　　　　　　B. 2 度 I 型 AVB

C. 2 度 II 型 AVB　　　　　　D. 3 度 AVB

E. 窦性心律不齐

32. 给下图作出正确的心电图诊断:

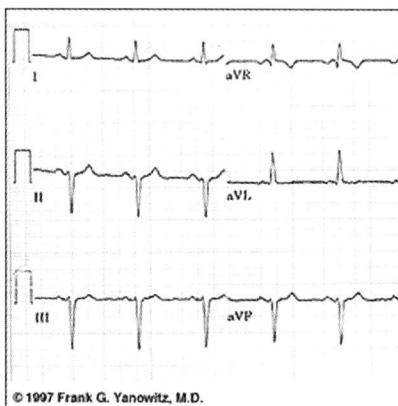

A. LBBB　　　　　　　　　　B. RBBB

C. LAFB　　　　　　　　　　D. RBBB + LAFB

E. RBBB + LPFB

33. 给下图作出正确的心电图诊断:

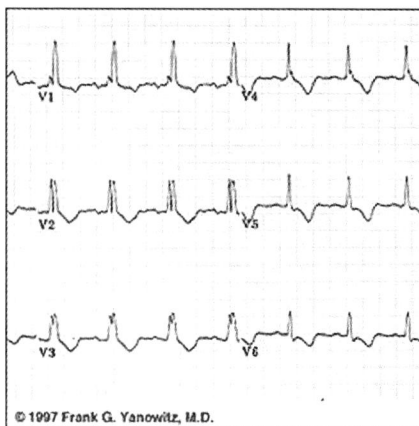

A. LBBB   B. RBBB

C. LAFB   D. RBBB + LAFB

E. RBBB + LPFB

34. 给下图作出正确的心电图诊断：

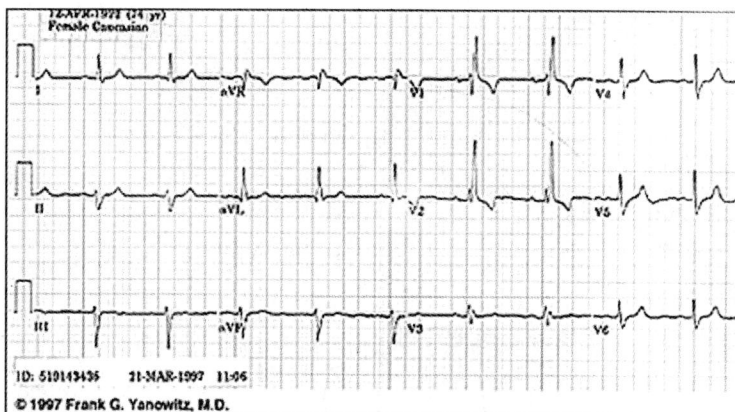

A. LBBB   B. RBBB

C. LAFB   D. RBBB + LAFB

E. RBBB + LPFB

35. 给下图作出正确的心电图诊断：

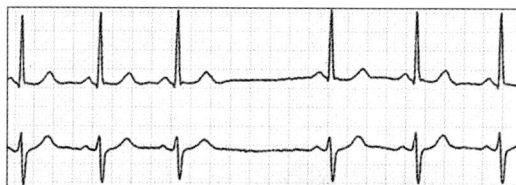

A. 窦性心律   B. 2 度 I 型 AVB

C. 2 度 II 型 AVB   D. 3 度 AVB

E. 窦房传出阻滞

36. 给下图作出正确的心电图诊断：

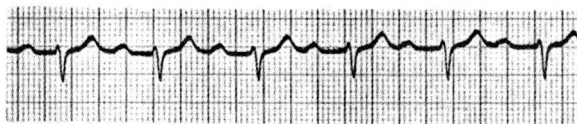

A. 1 度 AVB   B. 2 度 I 型 AVB

C. 2 度 II 型 AVB   D. 3 度 AVB

E. 窦房传出阻滞

37. 给下图作出正确的心电图诊断：

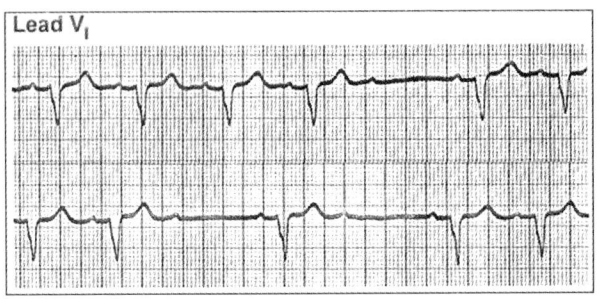

A. 1 度 AVB
B. 2 度 I 型 AVB
C. 2 度 II 型 AVB
D. 间歇性 3 度 AVB
E. 预激综合征

38. 给下图作出正确的心电图诊断：

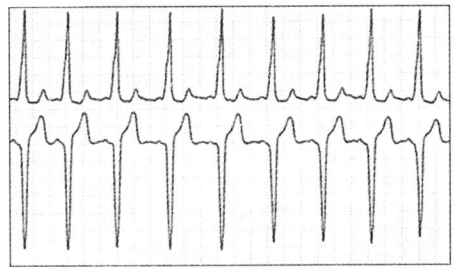

A. 1 度 AVB
B. 2 度 I 型 AVB
C. 2 度 II 型 AVB
D. 3 度 AVB
E. 预激综合征

39. 下列哪项关于心室肥厚（VH）的诊断标准的描述是正确的？
A. 满足了心室肥厚心电图标准的患者很可能患有心室肥厚
B. 没有满足心电图标准的患者没有心室肥厚
C. 应该使用康奈尔电压标准，因为它们的敏感性非常好
D. 心室肥厚的心电图标准敏感性和特异性至少 95%
E. 以上都不对

40. 左心房大的 P 波：
A. 振幅增加
B. 时间增加
C. 振幅和时间都增加
D. I 导联终末 P 波表现为负值
E. 以上都是

41. 右心室肥大（**RVH**）的心电图与下列哪种情况相似?

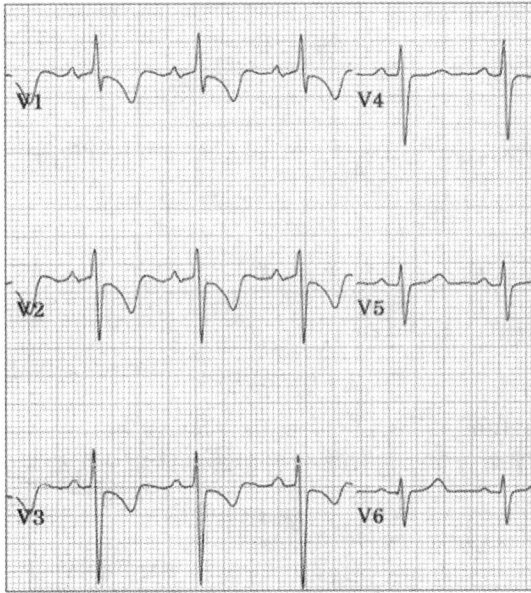

A. LBBB

B. AVB

C. 正后壁心肌梗死

D. LAFB

E. LPFB

42. 指出下列心电图的正确诊断:

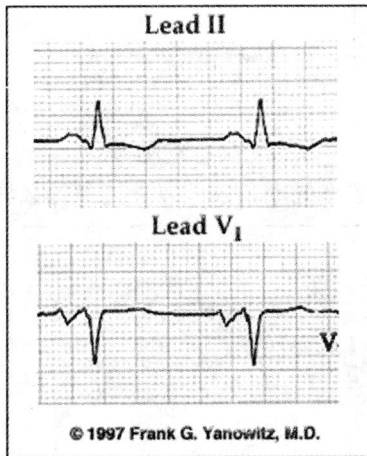

A. LVH

B. RVH

C. LAE(左心房大)

D. RAE（右心房大）

E. 双心房大

43. 什么是下列心电图的正确诊断？

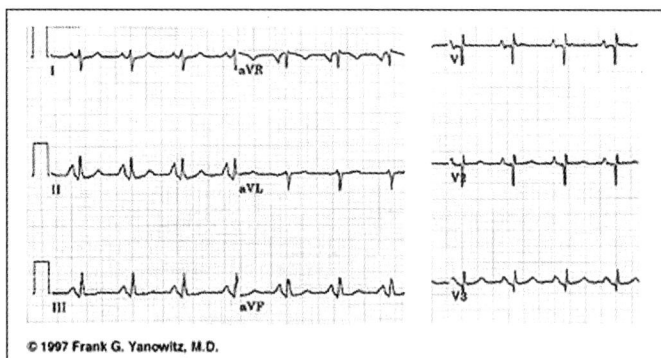

© 1997 Frank G. Yanowitz, M.D.

A. 左心房大　　　　　　B. 左心室肥大　　　　C. 双心房增大（BAE）

D. 左心房和左心室大　　E. 右心房和右心室大

44. 下面心电图中除了 1 度房室传导阻滞外还有什么异常？

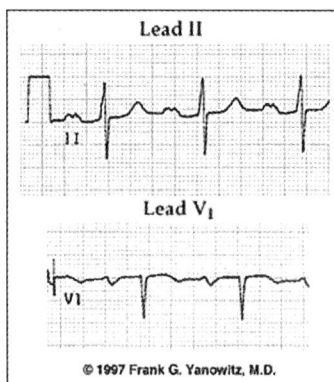

Lead II

Lead V₁

© 1997 Frank G. Yanowitz, M.D.

A. LAE　　　　　　　　B. RAE　　　　　　　C. LVH

D. RVH　　　　　　　　E. 双心室肥大

45. 下面心电图中除了室性期前收缩以外还有什么异常？

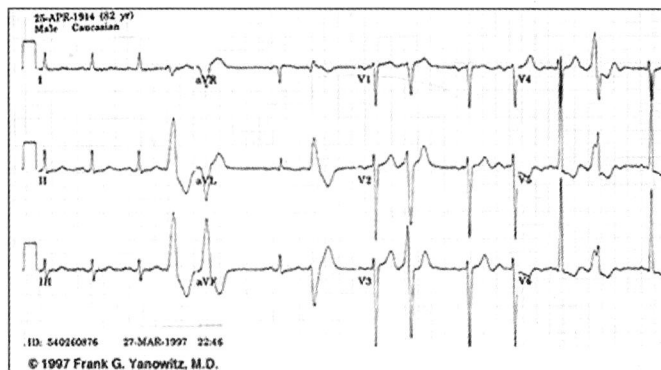

© 1997 Frank G. Yanowitz, M.D.

A. RAE   B. LAE   C. RVH

D. LVH   E. 双心室肥大

46. 给右图作出下列心电图的正确诊断：

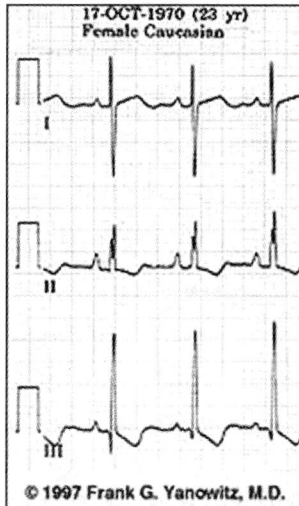

A. 电轴左偏和左心房大   B. 电轴右偏和右心房大

C. 左心房大和左心室大   D. 左心房大和右心房大

E. 电轴右偏和左心房大

47. 下面心电图最合适的诊断是什么？

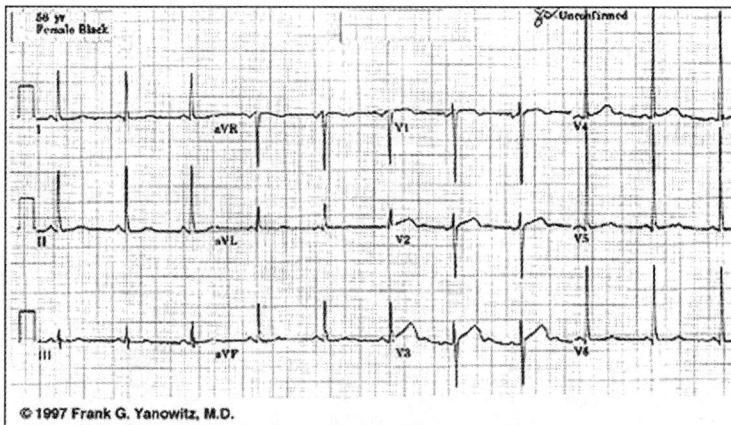

A. 左心室大   B. 右心室大

C. 左心房和左心室大   D. 右心房和右心室大

E. 以上都不是

48. 给出下列心电图的正确诊断：

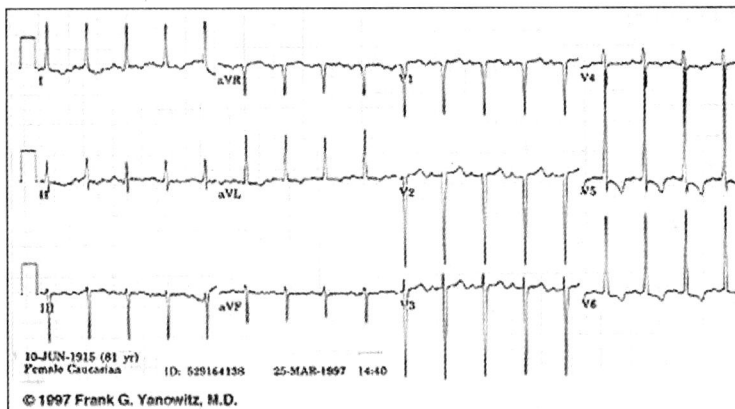

A. 左心房大   B. 右心房大

C. 左心室大伴压力负荷   D. 电轴右偏

E. 电轴左偏

49. 什么有助于鉴别正常的间隔 q 波和病理性 Q 波？

A. 宽度   B. 高度

C. 宽度和深度   D. QRS 电轴

E. 所涉及的心电图导联

50. 急性 ST 段抬高型心肌梗死（STEMI）的心电图表现中哪一项最先出现？

A. Q 波   B. ST 段抬高

C. 幅度和宽度均增加的超级性 T 波   D. Ⅰ 导联终末 P 波表现为负值

E. 以上都是

51. 给出下面心电图的正确诊断：

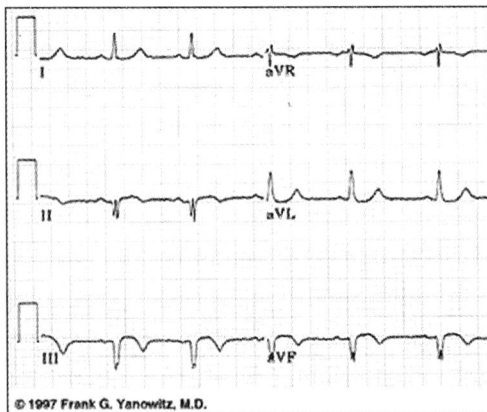

A. 前侧壁心肌梗死   B. 高侧壁心肌梗死

C. 正后壁心肌梗死   D. 下侧壁心肌梗死

E. 下壁心肌梗死

52. 给出下面心电图的正确诊断：

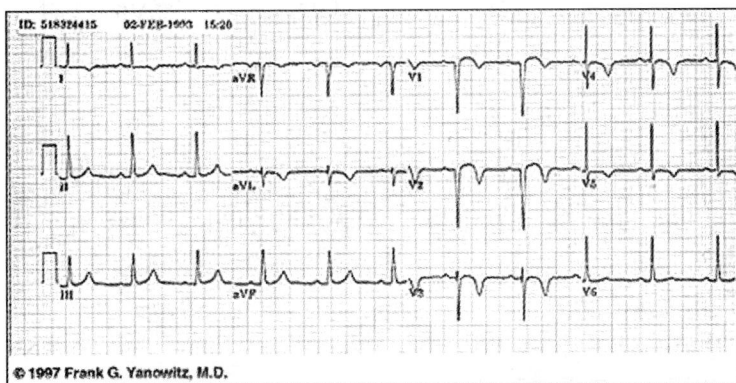

A. 前间壁心肌梗死   B. 前壁心肌梗死

C. 后壁心肌梗死   D. 后侧壁心肌梗死

E. 右心室心肌梗死

53. 给出下面心电图的正确诊断：

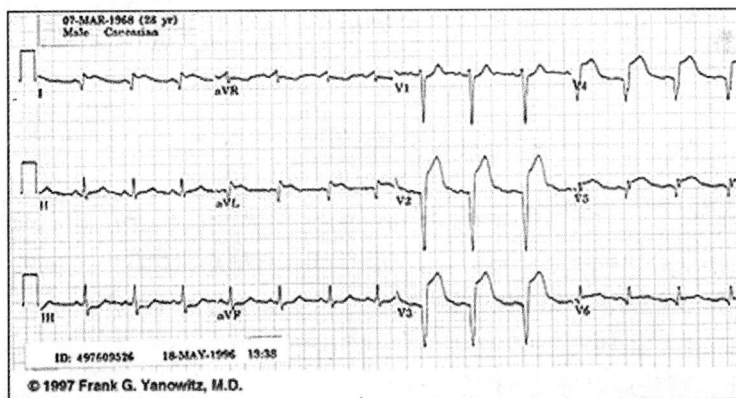

A. 正后壁心肌梗死   B. 广泛前壁/前侧壁心肌梗死

C. 下后壁心肌梗死   D. 后侧壁心肌梗死

E. 后侧壁心肌梗死 + LBBB

54. 给出下列心电图的正确诊断:

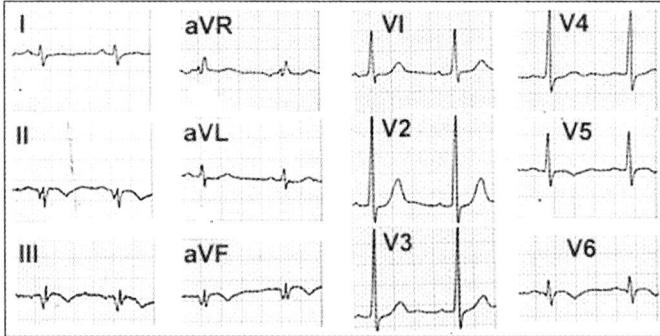

A. 下壁心肌梗死   B. 后壁心肌梗死

C. 下后壁心肌梗死   D. 前壁心肌梗死

E. 非 Q 波心肌梗死

55. 给出下面心电图的正确诊断:

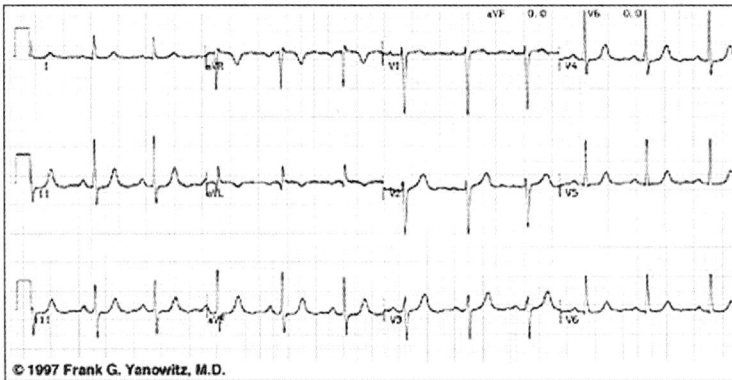

© 1997 Frank G. Yanowitz, M.D.

A. 高侧壁心肌梗死   B. 下壁心肌梗死

C. 下壁心肌梗死 + RBBB   D. 前侧壁心肌梗死

E. 正后壁心肌梗死

56. 下列哪些可以导致 ST 段压低?

A. 缺血   B. 过度换气

C. 心室肥大   D. 低血钾

E. 以上都是

57. 给出下面心电图的正确诊断：

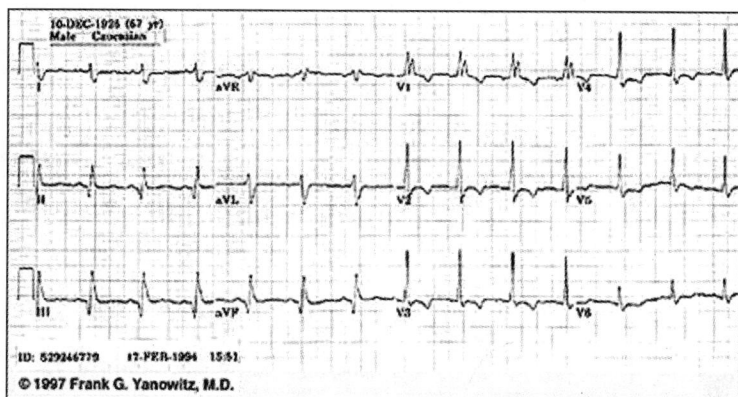

A. 下壁心肌梗死 + RBBB　　　　　B. 后壁心肌梗死 + LBBB

C. 下后壁心肌梗死　　　　　　　　D. 下后壁心肌梗死 + RBBB

E. 以上都不是

58. 给出下面心电图作出正确诊断：

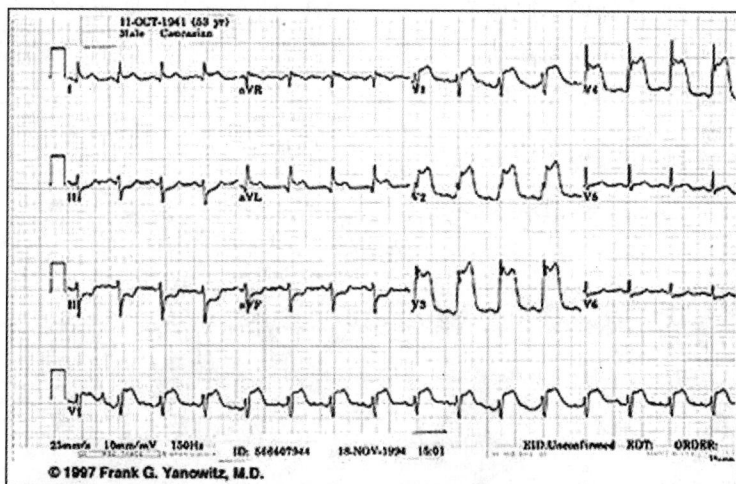

A. 非 Q 波心肌梗死　　　　　　　B. 急性前壁心肌梗死

C. 陈旧下壁心肌梗死　　　　　　　D. 前侧壁 + 高侧壁心肌梗死

E. 后侧壁心肌梗死

59. 正确描述右侧心电图：

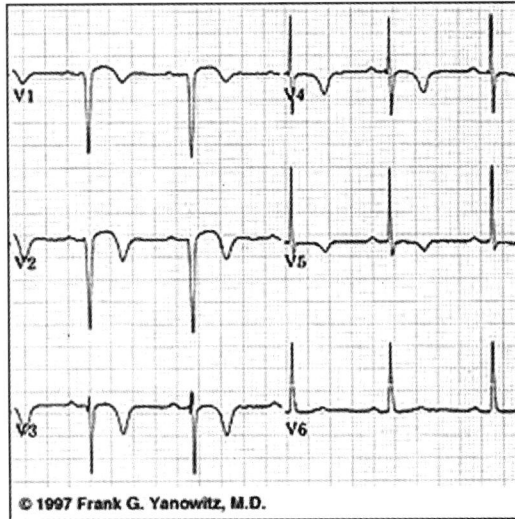

© 1997 Frank G. Yanowitz, M.D.

A. R 波进展不良

B. 弥漫性非特异性 ST – T 改变

C. 超急性期前间壁心肌梗死

D. 前间壁心肌梗死完全演变

E. 左心室肥厚伴压力负荷

60. 下面心电图中 ST – T 是：

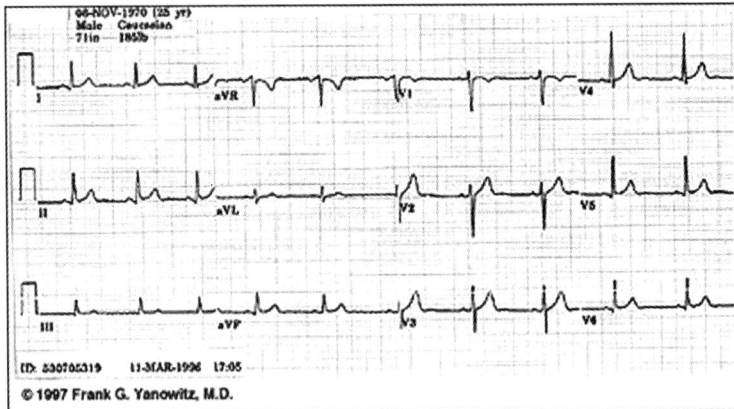

© 1997 Frank G. Yanowitz, M.D.

A. 原发性 ST – T 改变

B. 继发性 ST – T 改变

C. 非特异性 T 波改变

D. T 波异常倒置(aVR 和 V1)

E. 正常

61. 什么情况最容易产生下列心电图所见?

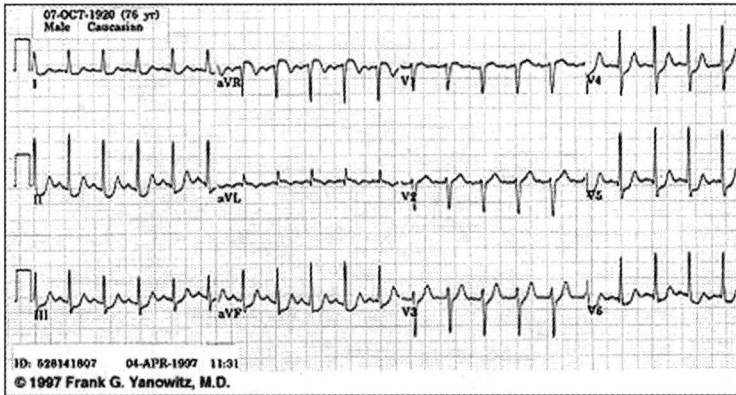

A. 心内膜下心肌缺血   B. 回旋支病变

C. 后壁透壁性损伤   D. 急性心包炎

E. 早期复极

62. 给出下列心电图的正确诊断:

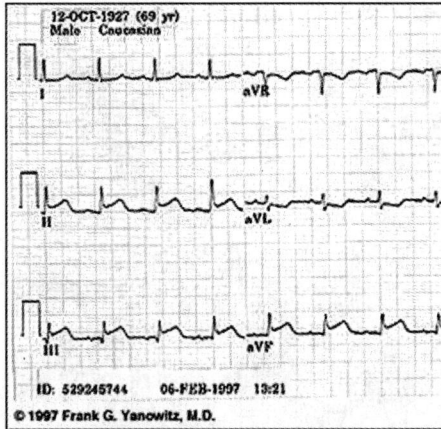

A. 正常变异的 ST 段抬高   B. 急性侧壁心内膜下缺血

C. 急性下壁透壁性缺血   D. 非特异性 ST - T 改变

E. 急性心包炎

63. 下列什么情况通常与原发性 ST - T 改变有关?

A. 束支阻滞   B. 房性期前收缩

C. 预激综合征(WPW)   D. 电解质紊乱

E. 分支阻滞

64. 下面心电图除了右束支阻滞外还有哪些异常？

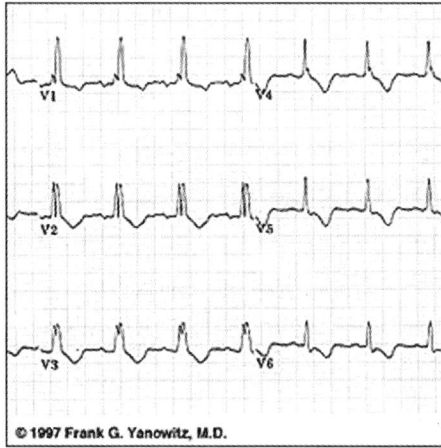

© 1997 Frank G. Yanowitz, M.D.

A. 原发性 ST – T 改变   B. 继发性 ST – T 改变

C. 前侧壁心肌梗死   D. LVH

E. RVH

65. 下面心电图代表了什么临床情况？

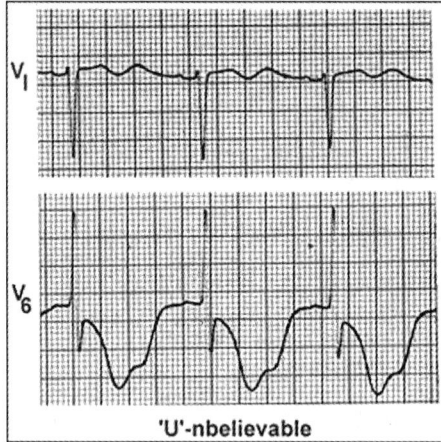

'U'-nbelievable

A. 急性心包炎   B. 蛛网膜下隙出血

C. 甲状腺功能低下   D. 主动脉狭窄

E. 这是正常心电图

66. 正常情况下哪些导联 U 波最清楚？

A. Ⅰ   B. V2, V3

C. Ⅱ, Ⅲ 和 aVF   D. aVL 或 aVR

E. Ⅰ 和 Ⅱ

67. 交界性心动过速时通常哪些导联容易见到倒置的 **P** 波？

A. Ⅰ，Ⅱ，Ⅲ   B. Ⅰ，Ⅱ，aVF

C. aVL，aVF，aVR   D. Ⅱ，Ⅲ，aVF

68. 下面心电图的主要异常是什么？

© 1997 Frank G. Yanowitz, M.D.

A. 电轴右偏   B. QRS 低电压

C. QT 间期延长   D. 高侧壁心肌梗死

E. T 波低平

69. 下面心电图显示 **LBBB** 伴有：

29-JUL-1907 (87 yr)
Female Caucasian
© 1997 Frank G. Yanowitz, M.D.

A. U 波异常   B. 原发性 ST – T 改变

C. T 波对称   D. 大 TU 融合波

E. 以上都是

70. 下面心电图最恰当的诊断应为：

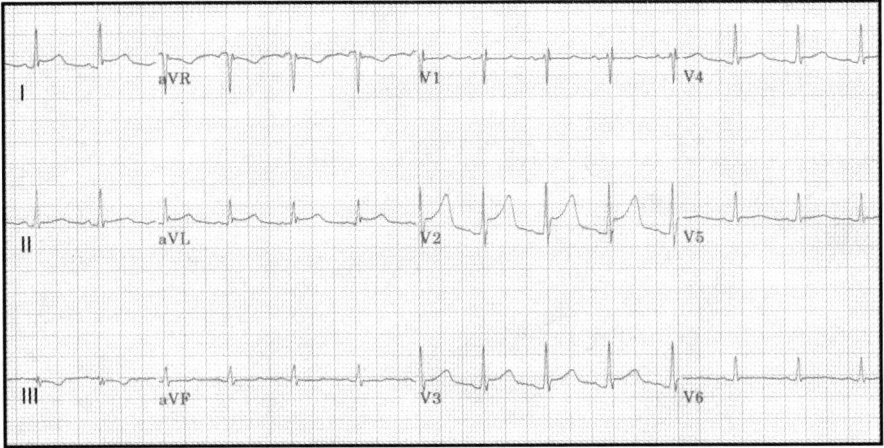

A. 急性前壁心肌梗死   B. 急性前壁＋高侧壁心肌梗死

C. 早期复极综合征   D. 急性心包炎

E. 以上都是

习题答案

1．B 2．D 3．A 4．B 5．B 6．D 7．C 8．C 9．D 10．A 11．E 12．C

13．C 14．C 15．E 16．E 17．A 18．B 19．E 20．D 21．A 22．D 23．B

24．C 25．E 26．B 27．E 28．A 29．A 30．B 31．B 32．C 33．B 34．D

35．E 36．A 37．C 38．E 39．A 40．B 41．C 42．C 43．E 44．A 45．D

46．B 47．A 48．C 49．C 50．C 51．E 52．C 53．C 54．C 55．A 56．E

57．D 58．B 59．D 60．E 61．A 62．C 63．D 64．A 65．C 66．B 67．B

68．C 69．B 70．D

答案 1—70 题详解：

1．B 是正确答案，房性期前收缩伴 RBBB 型差异性传导。注意宽大畸形的 QRS 波前有提前出现的房性期前收缩 P′波，第 1 个房性期前收缩下传未发生差异性传导，第 2 个房性期前收缩生了差异性传导是因为它前面的长－短周期导致的（Ashman 现象）。

2．D 是正确答案，"F"是融合波，是窦性下传兴奋了部分心室，室性期前收缩兴奋了部分心室，"F"的形态介于正常 QRS 波群和室性期前收缩的畸形波群之间；V1 导联的室性期前收缩是向上的正向波说明是从左后向右前除极，因此室性期前收缩是来源于左心室。

3．A 是正确答案，室性心动过速伴 2 : 1 传导阻滞。注意长的 RR 间歇正好是短的 RR 间歇的 2 倍，说明并不是每个室性异位搏动都能传出来。

4．B 是正确答案，舒张晚期的室性期前收缩通常与窦性同时兴奋心室，由于室性期前收缩出现的时间不同，与窦性发生融合的程度也不同，形态也不同。

5．B 是正确答案，2 度 Ⅱ 型 AVB，有的 P 波下传了，有的没下传。

6．D 是正确答案，"e"是交界性逸搏，"c"是窦性夺获。在任何一个节律中，如果有的间歇太长，就会产生逸搏。

7．C 是正确答案，窦性心律伴 1 度 AVB，偶发室性期前收缩。要"感谢"室性期前收缩，才让窦性 P 波暴露出来，否则融合在前面的 T 波里不容易被识别。

8．C 是正确答案，房性期前收缩未下传。注意很像 2 度 AVB，但是 P′波出现得早而且形态与正常窦性 P 波还是有区别的。

9. D 是正确答案,交界性逸搏终止了间歇。实际上在交界性逸搏的起始部可以看到窦性 P 波与其略有融合,显得交界性逸搏略增宽,容易误认为是室性逸搏。

10. A 是正确答案,2 度 Ⅱ 型 AVB。相邻的 PR 间期都是一致的,其后有 1 个窦性 P 波未下传,QRS 宽大提示合并束支阻滞。

11. 正确答案 E,电轴右偏 150°。Ⅱ 导联正向波与负向波几乎相等,为等电位导联,在 6 轴额面导联中与 aVL 正交(垂直相交),因此电轴方向不是 +150° 就是 −30°,那么通过 Ⅰ 和 Ⅲ 导联判断电轴右偏,所以是 +150°。

12. 正确答案 C,+30°。分析:Ⅲ 为等电位导联,与其正交的导联是 aVR 导联,指向 −150° 或 +30°,如果电轴是 −150° 指向 aVR,那么 aVR 应该以正向波为主(电流流向探测电极时为正向波),实际上 aVR 是负向波,所以电轴是另一端 +30°。

13. 正确答案 C,−30° 至 +90°。

14. 正确答案 C,电流方向从前向后。正常情况下。V1 和 V2 导联以负向波为主,说明电流是流向电极的相反方向。

15. 正确答案 E,V6 的电流方向与 Ⅰ 导联的相同,都是从左向右,正常情况下,两者都是正向波。

16. 正确答案 E,0°。aVF 接近等电位导联,正交导联是 Ⅰ 导联,电轴是 0° 或 180°,因为 Ⅰ 导联为正向波,所以电轴指向 Ⅰ 导联为 0°。

17. 正确答案 A,−75°。在这个心电图中看不到等电位导联,但是可以看到 Ⅰ 导联和 aVR 导联接近等电位导联,两者分别与 F 导联和 Ⅲ 导联正交,所以电轴是 −60° 和 −90° 之间或 +90° 和 +120° 之间,Ⅰ 导联和 aVR 导联为正向波为主,而 F 导联和 Ⅲ 导联是负向波,所以电轴是在 −60° 和 −90° 之间为 −75°。

18. 正确答案 B,aVF。通常 F 导联是正向波,F 电极在左足踝部,电流自上向下流向探测电极 F。

19. 正确答案 E,无法测量。因为 6 个导联都是等电位导联,是非常少见的正常变异。

20. 正确答案 D,+90°。等电位导联是 Ⅰ,正交 F 导联,指向 −90° 和 +90°,F 导联为正向波,所以电轴 +90°。

21. 正确答案 A,房性期前收缩。第 1 个房性期前收缩未产生差异性传导,第 2 个房性期前收缩前面有长短周期(Ashman 现象),所以产生 RBBB 型差异性传导。

22. 正确答案 D,室性期前收缩。提前出现的宽大畸形的 QRS 波群,不是室性期前收缩就是差异性传导。如何鉴别两者依据 3 点:①完全代偿间歇多为室性期前收缩；②宽大畸形的 QRS 前面是否有 P′或与 T 融合的 P′波，如果没有多为室性期前收缩；③本例中 V1 小"胖"r 波，以及从 r 的起点到 S 波下降支最低点 0.08 秒，多为室性期前收缩。

23. 正确答案 B，不完全代偿间歇。房性期前收缩两侧的 RR 间歇小于 2 个正常窦性的 RR 间歇，是因为房性期前收缩重置了窦房结时间。

24. 正确答案 C，心房纤颤。正常 P 波消失被小 f 波取代，RR 间距绝对不等（无规律的不规则）。本题图中第一条心电图看不清 f 波，第二条心电图中基线看上去像一个"老的锯齿"，与心房扑动的"新锯齿"相鉴别。

25. 正确答案 E，心房扑动 2∶1 阻滞。基线看上去像一个"新的锯齿"，RR 是规律的，心室率 150 次/min（心房率大约 300 次/min），这是最容易误诊为室上性心动过速的心电图，2 个 F 波中有 1 个下传到心室，另一个被房室结阻滞（因为房室结不应期还没过去）。

26. 正确答案 B，房室结折返性心动过速。房室结通常有双通道，当房性期前收缩产生时，如果快通道处在不应期而慢通道不应期已过，冲动就可以通过慢通道下传，当传到心室时快通道不应期已过，冲动又可以经快通道逆传到心房，然后再经慢通道下传形成折返。这是最常见的室上性心动过速。患者发作室上性心动过速时会描述心慌，心跳快。

27. 正确答案 E，加速性交界性心律。①QRS 前面没有 P 波后面可见倒置的 P′波；②QRS 无宽大畸形；③频率约 75 次/min，临床多见于缺血和药物作用。倒置 P′波可发生在 QRS 波前、中、后，如果频率 40 ~ 60 次/min 为交界性逸搏心律，60 ~ 100 次/min 称加速性交界性心律，如果大于 100 次/min，一般称交界性心动过速。

28. 正确答案 A，室性心动过速。这是来自右心室的室性心动过速，可以看到明显的房室分离和融合波（F）和窦性夺获（C），（﹡）来自于左心室。如果能看到室性融合波或窦性夺获者，大多为室性心动过速。

29. 正确答案 A，LBBB。①QRS 时间 >0.12 s；②Ⅰ导联和 V6 导联为单向波；③QRS 终末向量向左向后（Ⅰ，V1）。束支阻滞中 ST - T 方向与 QRS 的终末向量相反。

30. 正确答案 B，RBBB。V1 ~ V3 导联的 QRS 波为"M"型或 rSR′型且主波向上，V5，V6 导联 S 波增宽说明 QRS 终末向量向右前，左心室先除极右心室后除极，QRS 时间 >0.12 s。

31. 正确答案 B，2 度Ⅰ型 AVB。典型的文氏 3 原则：①PR 间期逐渐延长而 RR 间期逐渐缩短直到有 1 个 P 波脱落不能下传心室；②所产生的长 RR 间歇小于正常的 RR 间期的 2 倍；③间歇后的 RR 间期大于间歇前的 RR 间期。

32. 正确答案 C，LAFB。左前分支阻滞：①电轴左偏 ≥ - 30°（见Ⅰ，Ⅲ导联);②Ⅱ，Ⅲ和 aVF 导联 rS 型，S Ⅲ>S Ⅱ；③Ⅰ和/或 aVL 呈 qR 型；④QRS 无明显增宽。LAFB 是最常见的室内传导阻滞。

33. 正确答案 B，RBBB。特征详解见 30 题。但本例 V5 和 V6 导联可见原发性 ST – T 改变，RBBB 正常情况下 ST – T 初始方向与 QRS 终末向量方向相反，而本例相同。

34. 正确答案 D，RBBB + LAFB。这是最常见的室内双束支阻滞类型。RBBB 很容易辨认，V1 ~ V2 导联的"M"型 QRS 以及 V5 ~ V6 的宽 S 波；LAFB 的特征也符合，电轴左偏 –55°，Ⅱ导联，Ⅲ导联和 aVF 导联 rS 型，S Ⅲ>S Ⅱ，Ⅰ导联和（或）aVL 导联呈 qR 型。

35. 正确答案 E，窦房传导阻滞。①主要与 2 度Ⅱ型 AVB 鉴别：如果是 2 度Ⅱ型 AVB，P 波虽然不能下传心室没有 QRS 波，但是一定有 P 波，本例无 P 波说明心房没有兴奋，冲动在窦房结内被阻滞了；②与窦性心律不齐鉴别：窦性心律不齐的 RR 间期延长是渐进的，不是突然延长，而且长的 RR 间歇正好是短的 RR 间歇的 2 倍，说明这个冲动虽然在窦房结内被阻滞了，但是窦房结的规律没有乱。

36. 正确答案 A，1 度 AVB。正常 PR 间期 <0.20 s，本例 PR 约 0.30 s，所以是典型的 1 度 AVB。临床上多见于地高辛药物影响、缺血、心肌炎或迷走神经影响等。

37. 正确答案 C，2 度Ⅱ型 AVB。PR 无明显延长所以不是 1 度 AVB。2 度Ⅱ型 AVB 往往发生在双侧束支病变，2 个束支中往往有 1 个完全阻滞了（注意 V1 宽的负向 S 波说明是 LBBB），未下传的 P 波被阻滞在右束支上，表现为 2 度Ⅱ型的阻滞。

38. 正确答案 E，预激综合征。PR 间期缩短，可见 QRS 起始部的 delta 波，QRS 宽大畸形。

39. 正确答案 A，满足了心室肥厚心电图标准的患者很可能患有心室肥厚。临床上大约有一半心室肥厚的患者没达到心电图的诊断标准，因为左心室肥厚的心电图标准敏感性只有 50%。但是特异性高达 90%，所以满足了心室肥厚心电图标准的患者很可能患有心室肥厚。

40. 正确答案 B，时间增加。P 波时间 >0.12 s，而且 P 波有切迹。

41. 正确答案 C，正后壁心肌梗死。V1 导联的 R 波增高可见于许多情况，如正后壁心肌梗死、RBBB、WPW 和 RVH。有时人们称右心室肥厚为假性正后壁心肌梗死，两者 QRS 均表现为向前的向量，而 RBBB 往往在 V1 导联呈 rSR′ 型，WPW 可见短 PR 和 delta 波。

42. 正确答案 C，LAE（左心房大）。Ⅱ导联的 P 波 >0.12 s，V1 导联的 P 波负向波宽度 >0.04 s，深度 >0.1mv。

43. 正确答案 E，右心房大和右心室大。①右心房大：Ⅱ、Ⅲ、aVF 导联的 P

波振幅 >0.25mv；②右心室大：V1、V2 导联呈 Qr 型（或 rSR′），电轴右偏 +100°。

44. 正确答案 A，左心房大。详解见 42 题。

45. 正确答案 D，左心室大（LVH）。V2 导联的 S 波和 Ⅱ 导联的 R 波 >35mm（3.5mv）以及 ST - T 改变满足左心室大诊断标准。注意 V1 导联的 P 波提示左心房大。

46. 正确答案 B，电轴右偏和右心房大。电轴略大于 +90°，Ⅱ 导联的 P 波的振幅 >0.25mv 提示右心房大。本例是 1 个严重肺动脉高压的患者，同时存在右心室大，有些导联未提供。

47. 正确答案 A，LVH。Ⅱ 导联的 R 波 >20mm，V5 导联的 R 波 >30mm 满足左心室大诊断标准。

48. 正确答案 C，LVH 伴压力负荷。V2、V3、V5、V6 导联的 R 波电压明显增大，而且 ST - T 起始方向与 QRS 方向相反为左心室压力负荷表现，也称左心室肥厚兼劳损。

49. 正确答案 C，宽度和深度。病理性 Q 波时间 >0.04 s，深度 > QRS 波的 30%。

50. 正确答案 C，幅度和宽度均增加的超级性 T 波。超级性 T 波比 ST 段抬高较早出现，往往患者就医时已经看不到了。恢复期演变中 ST 段最先回落，然后 T 波逐渐倒置，Q 波可能长期存在。

51. 正确答案 E，下壁心肌梗死。这是典型的下壁梗死，Ⅱ、Ⅲ、aVF 导联明显的 Q 波和倒置的 T 波，ST 段未完全恢复到基线。注意每个导联都代表一个心脏的特定的部位。

52. 正确答案 A，前间壁心肌梗死。QRS 和 ST - T 都符合前间壁梗死的演变过程，注意 V3 ~ V5 的 T 倒置可能累及了前侧壁。为什么不是前壁梗死？前壁梗死一般 V1 没有 Q 波或 QS 波。

53. 正确答案 B，广泛前壁/前侧壁 MI。这是一例大面积心肌梗死的患者，涉及发生演变的导联越多梗死面积越大，预后越差。V2 - 6 和 I、aVL 都可见到明显的病理性 Q 波和 ST 段抬高，很可能是急性心肌梗死。

54. 正确答案 C，下后壁心肌梗死。下壁（膈面）导联 Ⅱ、Ⅲ、aVF 可见病理性 Q 波和倒置的 T 波，说明下壁有梗死；后壁梗死往往无病理性 Q 波，但是可以见到病理性 R 波（V1 ~ 3，R/S >1），应增加 V7 - 9 导联，注意和 RVH 鉴别。

55. 正确答案 A，高侧壁心肌梗死。I 和 aVL 可见到 Q 波，aVL 同时又有 T 波倒置和 ST 段略抬高，符合高侧壁梗死，如果不仔细观察容易漏诊。

56. 正确答案 E，以上都是。ST - T 的改变是非特异性的，许多情况都可以导致，比如地高辛作用，二尖瓣脱垂，中枢神经系统病变，甚至电极和皮肤接触不良也可导致。

57. 正确答案 D，后壁心肌梗死 + RBBB。本例中 Ⅱ、Ⅲ、aVF 的变化说明下壁梗死无疑，关键是合并 RBBB 还是合并后壁心肌梗死 + RBBB。如果合并一个单纯的 RBBB，V1 导联应为 rSR′，初始小 r 后面是大 R′，而本例初始 R 大于后面的 R′，提示同时合并后壁梗死，初始 R 与病理性 Q 具有等同意义。

58. 正确答案 B，急性前侧壁心肌梗死。V1 ~ V4 可见超急性 T 和 ST 明显抬高，提示急性前壁心肌梗死。虽然没有病理性 Q 波，也不能凭一次心电图就诊断非 Q 波梗死，因为随着心电图的演变，Q 波会出现。

59. 正确答案 D，前间壁心肌梗死完全演变。QS V1 ~ V2，qrS V3 以及 ST - T 的改变是前间壁梗死的完全演变。

60. 正确答案 E，正常。这是一个正常的心电图。正常 T 波是非对称的，上升支比较缓慢，倾斜度小，下降支速度快，倾斜度大，另外正常 T 波在 Ⅰ、Ⅱ 和 V4 - 6 导联永远都是直立的，aVR 是倒置的。V1 ~ V3 的 ST 段略抬高也是正常的。

61. 正确答案 A，心内膜下心肌缺血。虽然 ST - T 的改变是非特异性的，但是一旦出现就应该结合临床情况作出判断。心绞痛发作往往是心内膜下缺血表现为 ST 压低，不像 ST 段抬高可以对病变的冠状动脉做出定位，其他的选项应该有 ST 段抬高。

62. 正确答案 C，急性下壁透壁性缺血。本例是 1 个右冠状动脉痉挛引发的一过性 ST 段抬高，表现为 ST 段是直的或弓背向上的抬高往往是透壁性缺血，而心包炎或早期复极往往是弓背向下的 ST 抬高。Ⅱ、Ⅲ、aVF 的 ST 段抬高通常定位罪犯血管是右冠状动脉或者是左冠优势的回旋支动脉。

63. 正确答案 D，电解质紊乱。原发性 ST - T 改变是心脏整体或局部复极受到影响的结果，一般与心脏自身病变或异常有关；继发性 ST - T 改变是心室除极顺序改变导致的，如室性期前收缩、束支阻滞和 WPW 等。本例除 A 以外的其他选项均为继发性 ST - T 改变。

64. 正确答案 A，原发性 ST - T 改变。RBBB 的 ST 段方向正常情况下应该与 QRS 的终末向量相反，但是本例 V5，V6 的 ST 段与 QRS 的终末向量一致（都是负的）。V1 ~ V4 是正常 RBBB 表现，ST 段方向与 QRS 的终末向量相反。

65. 正确答案 B，蛛网膜下腔出血。看 V6 导联巨大的 TU 融合波和长 QT(U) 间期，其鉴别诊断包括：电解质紊乱（如低血钾），遗传性长 QT 间期综合征和药物作用（如奎尼丁）。

66. 正确答案 B。U 波最明显的导联是胸前导联尤其是 V2 和 V3，U 波明显增大最常见于低钾血症，在心肌缺血时 U 波可以倒置。

67. 正确答案 B。交界性心动过速的冲动前传可以到心室，逆传可以到心房，逆传是背离房室结向上兴奋心房（与正常窦性对心房除极方向相反）产生倒置 P′，

Ⅱ、Ⅲ、aVF 是显示正常窦性 P 波最明显的导联(P 为正值),因此也是显示逆传 P′(负值)最清楚的导联。

68. 正确答案 C。这道题中的关键词是"主要的",因为该心电图也存在电轴右偏、低电压,甚至 aVL 异常 Q 会误导为高侧壁心肌梗死(其实是电轴右偏导致),但是这些都没有 QT 延长重要,因为后者往往容易被忽略,而且通常会引起致命性心律失常(如尖端扭转型室性心动过速)。

69. 正确答案 B。本例是 LBBB 合并原发性 ST-T 改变,主要指 T 波方向与 QRS 后半部(终末向量)方向一致(都是正值或都是负值),见 Ⅰ,Ⅱ,Ⅲ,aVL,aVF 和 V3～V6 导联,很可能是一个心肌梗死。

70. 正确答案 D。特点是除了 aVR 外大多数导联 ST 段凹面向上抬高,没有对应的导联 ST 段压低(除外 aVR),与"早期复极"不同的是,T 波振幅通常较低,心率通常是增加的(100 次/min),Ⅰ、V2、V3 导联 PR 段压低,aVR 导联 PR 段抬高,提示心房损伤。当然,对心包炎的诊断还需要动态观察。

Thanks

I would like to thank Intermountain Healthcare for its support in allowing me to create this educational material to improve patient Care.

Frank G. Yanowitz, MD

致　谢

我非常感谢 Intermountain Healthcare 的大力支持并允许我完成这本教育资料，相信会造福于广大患者。

Frank G. Yanowitz 博士